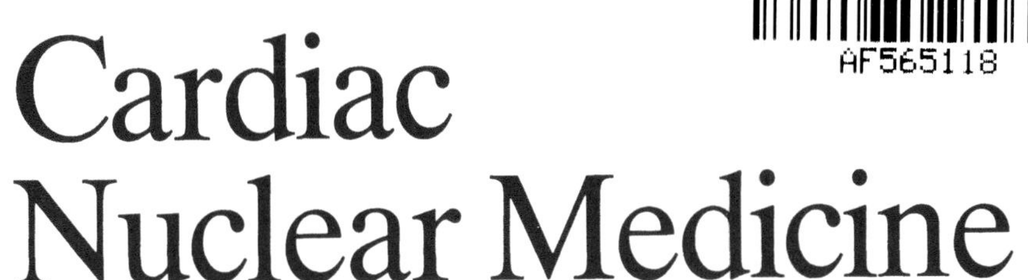

Cardiac Nuclear Medicine

Edited by

B. L. Holman

H. L. Abrams E. Zeitler

Contributors

W. E. Adam · F. Bitter · U. Buell · H.-J. Engel
H. Geffers · B. L. Holman · E. Kleinhans · A. Lenaers
P. R. Lichtlen · O. Nickel · N. Schad · M. Seiderer
M. Stauch · B. E. Strauer · A. Tarkowska · J. Wynne
J. S. Zielonka

With 47 Figures

Springer-Verlag Berlin Heidelberg GmbH

B. LEONARD HOLMAN, M.D.
Department of Radiology, Harvard Medical School, 25 Shattuck Street, Boston, MA 02115, USA

HERBERT L. ABRAMS, M.D.
Department of Radiology, Harvard Medical School, 25 Shattuck Street, Boston, MA 02115, USA

EBERHARD ZEITLER, Prof. Dr.
Klinikum Nürnberg, Radiologisches Zentrum, Flurstraße 17, D-8500 Nürnberg

This monograph comprises number 3 (Volume 2) of the Springer journal *CardioVascular Radiology*.

DOI 10.1007/978-3-642-67510-2

Library of Congress Cataloging in Publication Data. Main entry under title Cardiac nuclear medicine (Cardiovascular radiology, v 2, no 3) Bibliography· p Includes index 1. Radioisotopes in cardiology I Holman, Bruce Leonard II Abrams, Herbert L III Zeitler, Eberhard, 1930– IV Adam, W E. V Series RC683 5.R33C37 616 1′2′07575 79-26292

Originally published by Springer-Verlag Berlin Heidelberg New York 1979
MyCopy version of the original edition 1979

2127/3130-543210
www.springer.com/mycopy

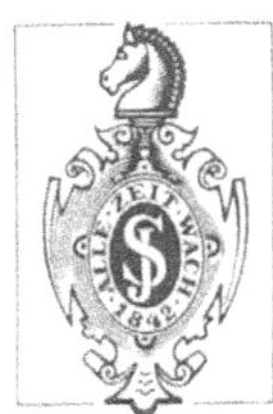

Preface

Cardiac nuclear medicine has grown dramatically over the past decade to the point where it is now an integral part of the routine diagnostic workup in patients with heart disease, particularly coronary artery disease. In no small part, this is the result of dramatic improvements in technology and the application of these improvements to the development and refinement of diagnostic techniques. In this book, authorities on cardiac imaging techniques provide an up-to-date description of the field, covering the clinical applicability, efficacy, and future potential of myocardial perfusion scintigraphy, quantitation of regional blood flow, assessment of ventricular performance, and detection of acute infarction using radiotracers. This book provides the physician involved in cardiac diagnosis with the background necessary to integrate the radiotracer method into his diagnostic armamentarium.

Boston, August 1979 B.L. Holman

Contents

Cardiac Nuclear Medicine: An Overview

B.L. Holman

Department of Radiology, Harvard Medical School and Peter Bent Brigham Hospital, Boston, Massachusetts, USA

The dramatic growth in cardiac nuclear medicine that has occurred over the past decade has resulted because of profound technological advances and the need for accurate noninvasive techniques to assess coronary artery perfusion and ventricular performance. With the development of high resolution scintillation cameras and highly sophisticated minicomputers, radionuclide techniques have taken their place alongside electrophysiologic and biochemical methodologies for the routine day-to-day assessment of patients with known and suspected cardiac disease.

Today, cardiac studies constitute between one-quarter and one-third of the imaging procedures performed in nuclear medicine. Patients are studied routinely under a number of physiologic and pharmacologic stresses, substantially enhancing the diagnostic potential of the techniques. Patients too sick to leave the coronary or intensive care units can be studied using mobile scintillation cameras and portable computer systems, expanding the applications of these techniques.

Cardiac nuclear medicine provides information comparable to that obtained with more invasive techniques, such as contrast left ventriculography, and also supplies data on regional cardiac function and perfusion that can be obtained by no other modality. The extension of these methods using three-dimensional reconstruction techniques and longitudinal tomography has remarkable potential for further developments in the field.

Instrumentation

The Single Probe Detector

The earliest probe detector for cardiovascular applications was the cloud chamber used by Blumgart and Weiss to study intravascular transit times in patients with congestive heart failure [1]. As ingenious as this system was, the radiochemistry and instrumentation was much too complicated for routine clinical applications.

The development of the sodium iodide crystal provided a simple, easy-to-use instrument for the measurement of radioactive transit. Radiocardiography using the sodium iodide crystal was first described by Prinzmetal in 1948 [2]. Subsequently, a number of investigators applied this technique successfully to the determination of end-diastolic and residual volumes of the whole heart and of the individual cardiac chambers [3–7]. Folse and Braunwald [8] used the scintillation probe for the measurement of the left ventricular ejection fraction after the ventricular injection of iodine-131-labeled diodrast.

The relative ease with which radiocardiography could be performed was not enough to overcome a number of important technical constraints. The first was the radiopharmaceutical. Iodine-131, usually in the form of ^{131}I-human serum albumin, results in a high radiation dose to the patient because of its relatively long half-life (eight days) and the associated nonpenetrating radiation due to beta decay. Thus, only small doses were administered to the patients, resulting in low count rates with correspondingly wide statistical fluctuations. With the introduction of short-lived nuclides such as technetium-99m and indium-113m in the early 1960s, these constraints were largely removed.

Limitations in instrumentation also hindered the clinical acceptance of radiocardiography. The sodium iodide detectors were used with analogue rate meters with long rate constants. As a result, the temporal resolution of the time-activity curves was between one-half and one second. The fluctuations in count rate that occur during a single cardiac cycle – data rich with information relating to blood volume changes during ventricular contraction – were averaged and lost to analysis. While cardiac output, pulmonary transit times, and pulmonary blood volume

Supported in part by USPHS grant HL17739. Dr. Holman is an Established Investigator of the American Heart Association

Address reprint requests to B. Leonard Holman, M.D., Department of Radiology, Harvard Medical School, 55 Shattuck Street, Boston, MA 02115, USA

could be measured despite these constraints, more important measurements of left ventricular function, such as ejection fraction, could not be determined without direct injection into the left ventricle.

High temporal resolution was possible with the development of digital and quick response analogue rate meters. With time constants of 0.05 seconds, changes in activity could be measured every 50 milliseconds.

The standard sodium iodide scintillation probe is 1–3 inches in diameter and between 1 and 2 inches in depth. The crystal is housed in either a cylindrical collimator [9, 10], a parallel hole collimator similar to the low-resolution, high-efficiency collimators used with scintillation cameras [9], or a converging collimator. The sodium iodide crystal is used with a high temporal resolution rate meter (10–50 msec). While the data can be displayed directly on a strip chart recorder, most systems now use a microprocessor for data acquisition and analysis. The time-activity curves are displayed on an oscilloscope, and the processed data is read out through a teleprinter or a console.

Scintillation Camera

The scintillation camera provides pictorial representation of the distribution of radioactivity. The Anger-type scintillation camera uses a single sodium iodide crystal detector 10 inches or more in diameter and between one-quarter and one-half inch in thickness. Photons are emitted in all directions from the point of disintegration. Photons that travel perpendicular to the crystal pass through the holes in the lead collimator and interact with the sodium iodide crystal. The position of the interaction within the crystal is detected by a bank of photomultiplier tubes that convert the electromagnetic energy to electrical current and determine the x and y position of the disintegration within the crystal. The resultant image is a map of the radioactive distribution within the patient. If sequential images are obtained, the regional change in radioactivity as a function of time can be measured.

A number of collimators have been suggested for radionuclide angiocardiography. The collimator selected for first-pass radionuclide angiography is usually constructed to maximize the counting rate and is therefore called a high-sensitivity collimator. Calculations from a first-pass study are based on five or six heartbeats at most, resulting in a count-limited study. The resolution in radionuclide imaging procedures is dependent primarily on total number of counts per image until a large enough activity has been recorded, at which point counting rate can be sacrificed for improved collimator resolution. First-pass studies do not collect enough counts to sacrifice them.

There is usually a tradeoff, however. For a given instrument, the higher the collimator sensitivity, the lower the resolution. The converging collimator is an exception, and it can also be used for first-pass studies. This collimator results in both high count rates and excellent spatial resolution. It is used with large field of view scintillation cameras. By and large, the parallel hole collimator is superior to a converging collimator because the efficiency of the crystal (the percent of counts recorded/the number of disintegrations) is uniform across the face of the crystal with the former but not the latter. The converging collimator also results in spatial distortions that affect geometric measurement.

Because of the increased counting efficiency of the newer generation of gamma cameras, a relatively high resolution collimator can be used for equilibrium studies without unduly extending the length of the procedure. In such studies, the apex of the heart is tilted toward the sternum in man, and the left atrium is behind the base of the left ventricle. If a straight bore parallel hole collimator were placed parallel to the chest, the left atrium would be superimposed on the left ventricle, and the left ventricle would appear foreshortened. This problem is overcome by using a 30° caudal tilt or by using a slant hole, straight bore collimator with a built-in 30° caudal tilt. Images obtained with this collimator in the left anterior oblique projection separate the left atrium from the left ventricle and view the ventricle normal to its long axis, eliminating the overlap of the apex onto the base that occurs in the standard left anterior oblique projection using a collimator with holes perpendicular to the detector [11].

The multicrystal camera is particularly well suited for first-pass studies in which high count rates are needed. The dead time determines the maximum count rate that can be accurately recorded by a gamma camera. When the activity is high, counts may not be recorded if the crystal has not fully recovered from the last disintegration. The higher the activity, the more counts lost and the less linear the relation between recorded counts and activity. Since the multicrystal camera is made up of 294 crystals, higher count rates can be acquired before any single crystal becomes saturated. Collimators for this camera are designed to take advantage of the camera's high count rate capabilities; 200,000 to 300,000 counts per second can be recorded with standard doses of currently available radiopharmaceuticals. The multicrystal camera uses a thin collimator with one hole per crystal to achieve its high count rate capability. Since each crystal within the detector acts as a single probe, the resolution of the camera is limited by the size of each detector (0.8 × 0.8 cm). While the resolution of the resultant dynamic image is poor, the global and regional information these studies provide is adequate for most clinical applications. Commercial models of this camera are not well suited for equilibrium studies, and portable versions are not available at the time of this writing.

For myocardial perfusion studies with thallium-201, a scintillation camera with high spatial resolution for the low photon energies of the thallium-201 characteristic x-rays is required. Collimator and imaging characteristics are discussed in the article "Quantitative Assessment of Thallium-201 Images" by U. Buell et al. later in this publication.

The Computer

Computer processing is essential with radionuclide angiography and reconstruction tomography and is helpful for myocardial perfusion with thallium-201. The combination of spatial and temporal information results in a large mass of data to be acquired and processed. While equilibrium radionuclide angiocardiograms were initially performed without the aid of a computer, the full potential of the technique requires at least some computer processing.

There are three types of computers available for data acquisition and analysis: (1) the general purpose digital minicomputer, (2) the special purpose minicomputer, and (3) the special purpose microprocessor. The most expensive and most flexible is the general purpose minicomputer. Its advantages are that special acquisition and processing programs can be written by the user and that a wide range of peripheral storage and display devices can be purchased as needed. This approach is most appealing in an environment where newer techniques are being developed and the possibility of unexpected changes is greatest. The disadvantages of the general purpose minicomputer are that an on-site computer programmer is required to take advantage of the programming capabilities and to manage the system. Because the computer manufacturer and the camera manufacturer are usually different, the resultant hybrid camera-computer system may have unforeseen servicing and engineering problems.

The special purpose minicomputer is built specifically for nuclear medicine functions and may be manufactured or sold by the camera manufacturers themselves. Programs are supplied by the manufacturer, and capabilities for user programming may be limited. The systems are relatively easy to use and less expensive than the general purpose computer. If the user cannot program the computer, he is at the mercy of the manufacturer for the development of programs to perform newer techniques as they are introduced.

Finally, the microprocessor is a relatively inexpensive data processing component that allows the user a limited data analysis and processing capability. Although it is the cheapest alternative, it is the least flexible and the most vulnerable of the three to obsolescence.

Radiopharmaceuticals

The primary requirement of a radiopharmaceutical for first-pass radionuclide angiocardiography is that it remain intravascular during its first passage through the right and left heart phases. The second requirement is that the radionuclide have satisfactory physical properties with respect to the instrumentation being used.

The radionuclide which has replaced iodine-131 for virtually all phases of radionuclide angiocardiography is technetium-99m. It has a six-hour half-life, a photon energy of 140 keV, and minimal nonpenetrating radiation. It can be labeled with a fairly large number of pharmaceuticals, a requirement that is particularly important for equilibrium studies. While pertechnetate leaks out rapidly into the extracellular space with an intravascular half-life of approximately one hour, it does remain intravascular during the first intravascular transit. Because the tracer need be intravascular only during its first transit, technetium-99m pertechnetate can be used for first-pass studies. Since ^{99m}Tc-pertechnetate ($^{99m}TcO_4^-$) is the chemical form of ^{99m}Tc after elution from the ^{99}Mo-^{99m}Tc generator, it is the most readily available and most inexpensive of the technetium-99m pharmaceuticals.

The major disadvantage of ^{99m}Tc is its long half-life relative to the time of the procedure. After intravenous injection, the material remains in the intravascular and extracellular space, precluding serial studies. Only two or three studies are possible within a six-hour period. As a result, evaluation in multiple projections or after multiple physiologic or pharmacologic interventions is not possible.

One approach to increasing the number of serial studies is the use of ^{99m}Tc-sulfur colloid, a radiopharmaceutical that is extracted by the reticuloendothelial system. The pharmaceutical is extracted primarily by the liver and spleen within several minutes after intravenous injection [12]. The disadvantage of this approach is the resultant high radiation dose to the bone marrow. Approximately 5% of the dose is sequestered by the bone marrow, the most radiosensitive of the body's tissues. ^{99m}Tc-pyrophosphate is an attractive alternative on the coronary care unit. Acute infarct scintigraphy can be performed 90 minutes after the initial first-pass study. Thus, two studies can be performed after the injection of a single radiopharmaceutical. ^{99m}Tc-DTPA (diethylene triamine pentaacetic acid) has also been suggested for first-pass studies since the blood clearance of this radiopharmaceutical is more rapid than that of ^{99m}Tc-pertechnetate, reducing the whole body radiation dose and, more important, shortening the time between sequential studies [13].

The development of short-lived radionuclides such as tantalum-178 ($t_{1/2}=9$ minutes) will increase the flexibility of this technique [14]. ^{178}Ta is obtained from a ^{178}W-^{178}Ta generator and can be imaged with a multicrystal camera or an Anger camera and pinhole collimator.

Indium-113m is a short-lived radionuclide that can be used with single probe radiocardiography. It has a half-life of 100 minutes and a photon energy of 363 keV. Because its photon energy is high, tissue absorption is minimal, and because its half-life is short, studies can be repeated at three to four hour intervals. Indium-113m is obtained from a ^{113}Sn-^{113m}In generator. Tin-113, the parent, has a half-life of 118 days. Indium-113m is not suitable for studies using the scintillation camera since the high photon energy results in low detector efficiency because of the thin crystals used in cameras and because of the relatively poor spatial resolution.

The radiopharmaceutical for equilibrium (ECG-gated) studies must remain in the intravascular space throughout the course of the study. If continual monitoring is anticipated, the radiopharmaceutical must remain within the intravascular space for at least one or two half lives. ^{99m}Tc-human serum albumin (HSA) and ^{99m}Tc-tagged red blood cells (RBCs) have been advocated for this purpose. ^{99m}Tc-HSA is less satisfactory for gated studies because: (1) there is proportionately more activity in the liver since the liver albumin space is larger than the intravascular space, and (2) the blood clearance of ^{99m}Tc-HSA is fairly rapid, precluding prolonged monitoring and restudies.

^{99m}Tc-RBCs have very slow blood clearance once the initial equilibration of the tracer has been reached. The red cells can be tagged in vivo by injecting 300–400 µg of stannous ion intravenously and injecting ^{99m}Tc-pertechnetate 15 minutes later. Approximately 60–80% of the pertechnetate labels the red blood cells, and the remainder is excreted through the kidneys. Equilibration is reached after five minutes. Since rapid renal clearance is a precondition for optimal studies, this technique is less satisfactory in patients with poor renal function, resulting in high background activity and poor target-to-background ratios. The primary advantage of this technique is the ease with which the red cells can be labeled. Recently, kits have been developed for the in vitro labeling of red cells. The major advantage of this approach is its high labeling efficiency (greater than or equal to 98%). While the technique takes more time than in vivo labeling, some kits now permit labeling in 15–30 minutes.

Myocardial perfusion scintigraphy is performed using potassium analogues as the radiotracer. The first potassium analogues available for human use had energies that were unsatisfactory for imaging with scintillation detectors [15–17]. Potassium-43 is the first of a number of potassium analogues that have physical characteristics that are at all compatible with external imaging [18]. While results with this agent have been promising, use of this radiotracer is still limited by its relatively long half-life (22.4 hours); by beta emission that results in a high absorbed dose to the patient; by highly energetic photons with a photopeak at 373 keV, which makes imaging with the gamma camera quite difficult; and by a highly abundant photopeak at 619 keV that results in substantial degradation of the image due to scatted radiation.

Other potassium analogues have been introduced recently, including cesium-129 [19], rubidium-81 [20], and thallium-201 [21]. All have physical characteristics that represent improvements over ^{43}K and are clearly superior to the first generation of potassium analogues.

Thallium-201, a metallic element with properties similar to potassium [22, 23], is the radiopharmaceutical of choice for myocardial perfusion scintigraphy. Blood clearance of thallium is nearly as rapid as that of potassium or rubidium, and the myocardial clearance is slower, giving a maximum heart-to-blood ratio at ten minutes. The distributions of thallium and rubidium throughout the left ventricle are quite similar. Thallium appears to concentrate in myocardium to a somewhat greater degree than potassium or rubidium [24].

In addition to biologic advantages over potassium and the other potassium analogues, this tracer has physical characteristics more ideally suited for imaging with scintillation camera systems [24]. While the gamma emission from ^{201}Tl is 135 and 165 keV, only 10% of disintegrations result in these gamma rays. Characteristic x-rays given off in the range of 69–83 keV, however, are quite useful for external imaging. While the use of this energy peak results in some loss of spatial resolution due to the difficulty of completely eliminating scattered radiation from the primary photopeak by pulse-height analysis, this energy range does permit imaging with scintillation cameras and enables greater resolution than is obtained with either ^{43}K, ^{81}Rb, or ^{129}Cs. The extraction of thallium by the myocardium is most likely due to activation of the sodium-potassium adenosine triphosphatase system. Thallium appears to bind at two sites on the enzyme system compared to one for potassium. This may account for the prolonged clearance of thallium from the myocardium [23].

When cyclotron-produced positron-emitting potassium analogues and positron imaging devices are used in perfusion scintigraphy, three-dimensional reconstruction of the heart is possible. The very short half-life of these agents also permits multiple studies under various stress states and frequent sequential examinations to follow the course of ischemia or infarction. One of these promising agents is rubidium-82, a positron emitter with a 75-second half-life [25]. Aside from the obvious advantages that result from its short half-life, this potassium analogue is the daughter of strontium-82, which has a 25-day half-life. Since strontium-82-rubidium-82 generator systems have been developed [26], the parent (^{82}Sr) can be stored for considerable periods and eluted whenever ^{82}Rb is needed for injection. While imaging with rubidium-82 is not possible with the gamma camera, high resolution scintiscans have been obtained in animal models when coincidence imaging is used with the positron camera [27].

A number of positron-emitting radiopharmaceuticals have been used in the evaluation of coronary artery disease. Ammonia ($^{13}NH_3$) has been used as a marker of myocardial perfusion, and a close correlation has been found between changes in size of the resultant perfusion defect and the clinical course of patients with acute infarction [28]. The fatty acid, palmitate, has been labeled with ^{11}C and has been used to assess infarction and myocardial metabolism (see "Emission Tomography of the Heart: Principles and Applications," by J.S. Zielonka and B.L. Holman).

The first successful ^{99m}Tc-labeled infarct-avid radiopharmaceutical was ^{99m}Tc-tetracycline [29, 30]. It suffered from several biologic characteristics that limited its clinical use. Blood clearance was slow, requiring delayed imaging, and its target-background ratio was relatively low. ^{99m}Tc-pyrophosphate proved a superior radiotracer for infarct detection, clearing rapidly from the blood and achieving infarct-to-normal-myocardium ratios of 15–20:1 [31]. Other tracers are sequestered in the acute infarct, but none have characteristics that are clearly superior to ^{99m}Tc-pyrophosphate. The mechanism of ^{99m}Tc-pyrophosphate and the structure: activity relationships involved in infarct binding of other tracers are discussed in the review "Myocardial Scintigraphy with Infarct-Avid Tracers" later in this publication.

Ventricular Performance

Ventricular performance is a prime factor in determining appropriate medical and surgical management in patients with coronary heart disease [32–35]. Left ventricular ejection fraction and regional wall motion are directly related to the clinical prognosis in patients with chronic coronary heart disease [32–34] and in patients after myocardial infarction [36, 37]. Invasive techniques provide reliable measurements of ejection fraction and regional wall motion [38]. These techniques, however, have limited applicability in clinical situations requiring serial evaluations of ventricular function and evaluation of critically ill patients. Radionuclide techniques are noninvasive, requiring only a peripheral intravenous injection, and offer distinct advantages over conventional invasive methods. The radionuclide techniques are safe and repeatable and do not induce measurable hemodynamic alterations [13]. Critically ill patients, too sick to be transported to the nuclear medicine clinical unit, can be studied at the bedside with mobile scintillation cameras and probe detectors, and thus hemodynamic measurements can be obtained at any location throughout the hospital.

There are two general types of radionuclide techniques for assessing ventricular performance. First-pass techniques measure indices of cardiac performance from the initial transit of the radiotracer through the heart. The technique and the clinical applications of first-transit studies are discussed by N. Schad and O. Nickel in their review "Assessment of Ventricular Function with First-Pass Angiocardiography". Equilibrium studies measure ventricular function using radiotracers that have reached equilibrium in the intravascular space. This technique and its advantages and disadvantages over first-pass techniques are reviewed by W.E. Adam et al. in their article "Equilibrium (Gated) Radionuclide Ventriculography".

Myocardial Perfusion Scintigraphy

The development of surgical and medical techniques for the treatment of coronary artery disease has dramatized the need for an objective measure of regional myocardial perfusion. Although the coronary arteriogram can provide precise definition of vessel morphology, the effect of a coronary artery lesion on tissue perfusion cannot be accurately determined by roentgenographic procedures [39]. Furthermore, objective screening procedures are needed to evaluate patients during the early stages of their disease, well before symptoms become severe enough to warrant catheterization.

Radionuclide techniques that assess regional myocardial perfusion provide information useful in the detection and evaluation of coronary artery disease and in the assessment of therapies aimed at limiting the degree of ischemia and the extent of tissue necrosis. Obtaining regional information is critical since coronary heart disease is a diffuse disease with areas of normal myocardium mixed in with severely diseased tissue. It is important to measure perfusion both at rest and during exercise or other stress-simulating states since perfusion may be normal at rest even in patients with severe coronary artery disease. It is also critical that these techniques assess myocardial blood flow directly, to determine the net effect of such factors as the extent and number of coronary artery lesions, the adequacy of collateral circulation, and the presence of nonviable tissue in coronary artery disease.

The radiopotassium distribution will reflect blood flow accurately only if the extraction fraction remains the same at different flows. This is indeed the case over a relatively wide range of blood flow values. Regional myocardial perfusion is systematically underestimated by radiopotassium uptake at high flow values [40, 41]; however, conversely, at very low flow rates (less than 10% of normal), radiopotassium analogues overestimate blood flow, probably because myocardial extraction increases as flow rates approach zero [42].

Another factor that affects the distribution of potassium is the integrity of the cell membrane adenosine triphosphatase system, which maintains transmembrance electrochemical gradients of sodium and potassium [43, 44]. Alterations to the system should theoretically result in decreased efficiency of potassium-43 extraction during exercise-induced angina. For example, in the presence of severe regional hypoxia with adequate perfusion, the concentration of radiocesium is decreased [45]. In the presence of decreased flow, however, the effect of increased extraction efficiency more than compensates for any transient alterations in the active transport or membrane permeability of the radiotracer. The clinical application of myocardial perfusion scintigraphy in the assessment of coronary artery disease is described in detail in the contributions of U. Buell et al. "Quantitative Assessment of Thallium-201 Images" and of A. Lenaers, "Thallium-201 Myocardial Perfusion Scintigraphy during Rest and Exercise" in this edition.

Many of the problems associated with conventional two-dimensional imaging are overcome with tomography, with either positrons or thallium-201. The current state of the art of reconstruction tomography is described by J.S. Zielonka and B.L. Holman in "Emission Tomography of the Heart: Principles and Applications" in this publication.

More invasive techniques have been developed to assess quantitatively the significance of coronary artery lesions found at coronary angiography. These techniques suffer from the limitation of having to be performed during or after coronary angiography; they are thus of limited use in the serial evaluation of patients with coronary artery disease. Nevertheless, these techniques provide a quantitative measure of blood flow that is an important complement to the data obtained by coronary arteriography. Flow may be assessed both at rest and following intervention to determine regional myocardial blood flow distal to coronary artery lesions; thus, the hemodynamic significance of the lesions can be determined. It may also be possible to distinguish myocardial segments that are irreversibly scarred from prior infarcts.

The inert gas washout method provides a quantitative measure of specific flow (ml/min/100 g). The inert gas dissolved in saline is injected directly into the coronary artery. Once the tracer has diffused into the tissue, the organ is perfused by tracer-free blood, thus setting up a concentration gradient between the tissue and blood. Since the tracer is not diffusion-limited, the rate at which the tracer diffuses back into the blood depends on the flow rate through the tissue and the solubility partition coefficient between blood and tissue. The more rapid the flow rate, the more rapid the clearance or washout from the tissue. The application of this technique to our understanding of the changes in coronary blood flow resulting from coronary artery pathology is reviewed in the article "Assessment of Regional Myocardial Blood Flow Using the Inert Gas Washout Technique," by P.R. Lichtlen and H.-J. Engel.

This review issue of *Cardiovascular Radiology* provides a general overview of cardiac nuclear medicine and may be particularly useful for the reader who has not as yet incorporated cardiac nuclear medicine techniques into his diagnostic armamentarium. The very excellent contributions to this issue by my colleagues should help put cardiac nuclear medicine in proper perspective as a revolutionary modality in the noninvasive evaluation of cardiac disease.

References

1. Blumgart, H.L., Weiss, S.: Studies on the velocity of blood flow: II. The velocity of blood flow in normal resting individuals, and a critique of the method used. J. Clin. Invest. 4:15–32, 1927
2. Prinzmetal, M., Corday, E., Bergman, H.C., Schwartz, L., Spritzler, R.J.: Radiocardiography: A new method for studying the blood flow through the chambers of the heart in human beings. Science 108:340–341, 1948
3. Donato, L.: Radiocardiographic determinations in man of diastolic and residual blood volumes. Minerva Nucl. 2:12–14, 1958
4. Thode, H.G., Donato, L.A., Debus, G.H., Nace, P.F., Jaimet, C.H.: Inhalation radiocardiography. Ann. Int. Med. 48:537–561, 1958
5. Cournand, A., Donato, L. Durand, J. Rochester, D.F., Parker, J.O., Harvey, R.M., Lewis, M.L.: Separate performance of both ventricles in man during the early phase of exercise, as analyzed by the method of selective radiocardiography. Trans. Assoc. Am. Physicians 73:283–296, 1960
6. Lammerant, J., Sprumont, P., DeVisscher, M.: Enregistrement du flot sanguin intracardiac chez l'homme par une methode de dilution d'isotopes radioactifs. Arch. Int. Physiol. 64:65–71, 1956
7. MacIntyre, W.J., Pritchard, W.H., Moir, T.W.: The determination of cardiac output by the dilution method without arterial sampling. Circulation 18:1139–1146, 1958
8. Folse, R., Braunwald, E.B.: Determination of fraction of left ventricular volume ejected per beat and of ventricular end-diastolic and residual volumes. Circulation 25:674–685, 1962
9. Bacharach, S.L., Green, M.V., Borer, J.S., Ostrow, H.G., Redwood, D.R., Johnston, G.S.: ECG-gated scintillation probe measurement of left ventricular function. J. Nucl. Med. 18:1176–1183, 1977
10. Steele, P., Van Dyke, D., Trow, R.S., Anger, H.O., Davies, H.: A simple and safe bedside method for serial measurement of left ventricular ejection fraction, cardiac output, and pulmonary blood volume. Br. Heart J. 36:122–131, 1974
11. Parker, J.A., Uren, R.F., Jones, A.G., Maddox, D.E., Zimmerman, R.E., Neill, J.M., Holman, B.L.: Radionuclide left ventriculography with the slant hole collimator. J. Nucl. Med. 18:848–851, 1977
12. Marshall, R.C., Berger, H.J., Costin, J.D., Freedman, G.S., Wolberg, J., Cohen, L.S., Gottschalk, A., Zaret, B.L.: Assessment of cardiac performance with quantiative angiocardiography. Circulation 56:820–829, 1977
13. Ashburn, W.L., Schelbert, H.R., Verba, J.W.: Left ventricular ejection fraction: A review of several radionuclide angiographic approaches using the scintillation camera. Prog. Cardiovasc. Dis. 20:267–284, 1978
14. Holman, B.L., Harris, G.I., Neirinckx, R.D., Jones, A.G., Idoine, J.: Tantalum-178 – a short-lived nuclide for nuclear medicine: Production of the parent ^{178}W. J. Nucl. Med. 19:510–513, 1978
15. Bennett, K.R., Smith, R.O., Lehan, P.H., Hellems, H.K.: Correlation of myocardial ^{42}K uptake with coronary arteriography. Radiology 102:117–124, 1972
16. Carr, E.A., Jr., Beierwaltes, W.H., Wegst, A.V., Bartlett, J.D., Jr.: Myocardial scanning with rubidium-86. J. Nucl. Med. 3:76–82, 1962
17. Carr, E.A., Jr., Walker, B.J., Bartlett, J., Jr.: The diagnosis of myocardial infarcts by photoscanning after administration of cesium^{131} (abstract). J. Clin. Invest. 42:922, 1963
18. Hurley, P.J., Cooper, M., Reba, R.C., Poggenburg, K.J., Wagner, H.N., Jr.: ^{43}KCl: A new radiopharmaceutical for imaging the heart. J. Nucl. Med. 12:516–519, 1971
19. Romhilt, D.W., Adolph, R.J., Sodd, V.C., Levenson, N.I., August, L.S., Nishiyama, H., Berke, R.A.: Cesium-129 myocardial scintigraphy to detect myocardial infarction. Circulation 48:1242–1251, 1973
20. Martin, N.D., Zaret, B.L. McGowan, R.L., Wells, H.P., Jr., Flamm, M.D.: Rubidium-81: A new myocardial scanning agent. Radiology 111:651–656, 1974
21. Lebowitz, E., Greene, M.W., Bradley-Moore, P., Atkins, H., Ansari, A., Richards, P., Belgrave, E.: ^{201}Tl for medical use (abstract). J. Nucl. Med. 14:421–422, 1973
22. Gehring, P.J., Hammond, P.B.: The interrelationship between thallium and potassium in animals. J. Pharmacol. Exp. Ther. 55:187–201, 1967
23. Britten, J.S., Blank, M.: Thallium activation of the (Na^+-K^+)-activated ATPase of rabbit kidney. Biochim. Biophys. Acta 159:160–166, 1968
24. Strauss, H.W., Harrison, K., Langan, J.K., Lebowitz, E., Pitt, B.: Thallium-201 for myocardial imaging. Relation of thallium-201 to regional myocardial perfusion. Circulation 51:641–645, 1975
25. Budinger, T.F., Yano, Y., Hoop, B.: A comparison of $^{82}Rb^+$ and $^{13}NH_3$ for myocardial positron scintigraphy. J. Nucl. Med. 16:429–431, 1975
26. Yano, Y., Anger, H.O.: Visualization of heart and kidneys in animals with ultrashort-lived ^{82}Rb and the positron scintillation camera. J. Nucl. Med. 9:413–415, 1968
27. Vokelman, J., Van Dyke, D., Yano, Y.: Myocardial scanning with rubidium-82. Stokely Laboratory Reports 775, 1972
28. Walsh, W.F., Fill, H.R., Harper, P.V.: Nitrogen-13-labeled ammonia for myocardial imaging. Sem. Nucl. Med. 7:59–66, 1977
29. Holman, B.L., Dewanjee, M.K., Idoine, J., Fliegel, C.P., Davis, M.H., Treves, S., Eldh, P.: Detection and localization of experimental myocardial infarction with ^{99m}Tc-tetracycline. J. Nucl. Med. 14:595–599, 1973
30. Holman, B.L., Lesch, M., Zweiman, F.G., Temte, J., Lown, B., Gorlin, R.: Detection and sizing of acute myocardial infarcts with ^{99m}Tc(Sn)tetracycline. N. Engl. J. Med. 291:159–163, 1974
31. Bonte, F.J., Parkey, R.W., Graham, K.D., Moore, D., Stokely, E.M.: A new method for radionuclide imaging of myocardial infarcts. Radiology 110:473–474, 1974
32. Cohn, P.F., Gorlin, R., Cohn, L.H., Collins, J.J., Jr.: Left ventricular ejection fraction as a prognostic guide in surgical treatment of coronary and valvular heart disease. Am. J. Cardiol. 34:136–141, 1974
33. Nelson, G.R., Cohn, P.F., Gorlin, R.: Prognosis in medically treated coronary artery disease: The value of ejection fraction compared with other measurements. Circulation 52:408–412, 1975
34. Feild, B.J., Russell, R.O., Jr., Dowling, J.T., Rackley, C.E.: Regional left ventricular performance in the year following myocardial infarction. Circulation 46:679–689, 1972
35. Watson, L.E., Dickhaus, D.W., Martin, R.H.: Left ventricular aneurysm: Preoperative hemodynamics, chamber volume, and results of aneurysmectomy. Circulation 52:868–873, 1975
36. Schelbert, H.R., Henning, H., Ashburn, W.L., Verba, J.W., Karliner, J.S., O'Rourke, R.A.: Serial measurements of left ventricular ejection fraction by radionuclide angiography early and late after myocardial infarction. Am. J. Cardiol. 38:407–415, 1976
37. Rigo, P., Murray, M., Strauss, H.W., Taylor, D., Kelly, D., Weisfeldt, M., Pitt, B.: Left ventricular function in acute myo-

cardial infarction evaluated by gated scintiphotography. Circulation 50:678–684, 1974
38. Karliner, J.S., Gault, M.D., Eckberg, D., Mullins, C.B., Ross, J., Jr.: Mean velocity of fiber shortening: A simplified measure of left ventricular myocardial contractility. Circulation 44:323–333, 1971
39. Abrams, H.L., Adams, D.F.: The coronary arteriogram: Structural and functional aspects. N. Engl. J. Med. 281:1276–1285, 1969
40. Becker, L., Ferreira, R., Thomas, M.: Comparison of ^{86}Rb and microsphere estimates of left ventricular bloodflow distribution. J. Nucl. Med. 15:969–973, 1974
41. Moir, T.W.: Measurement of coronary blood flow in dogs with normal and abnormal myocardial oxygenation and function: Comparison of flow measured by a rotameter and by Rb^{86} clearance. Circ. Res. 19:695–699, 1966
42. Love, W.D., Burch, G.E.: Influence of the rate of coronary plasma flow on the extraction of Rb-86 from coronary blood. Circ. Res. 7:24–30, 1959
43. Case, R.B.: Ion alterations during myocardial ischemia. Cardiology 56:245–262, 1971
44. Parker, J.O., Chiong, M.A., West, R.O., Case, R.B.: The effect of ischemia and alterations of heart rate on myocardial potassium balance in man. Circulation 42:205–217, 1970
45. Levenson, N.I., Adolph, R.J., Romhilt, D.W., Gabel, M., Sodd, V.C., August, L.S.: Effect of myocardial hypoxia and ischemia on myocardial scintigraphy. Am. J. Cardiol. 35:251–257, 1975

Assessment of Ventricular Function with First-Pass Angiocardiography

N. Schad and O. Nickel

Department of Radiology, City Hospital, Passau, FRG

Assessment of ventricular function is important in the evaluation of patients with known or suspected coronary artery disease. The rapid deterioration in contractility in myocardial segments with inadequate coronary blood flow leads to regional abnormalities of ventricular wall contraction. Because of the segmental reduction in wall shortening, there is diminished force for regional ejection of blood, and overall ventricular performance is deprived of the contribution of the involved myocardium.

Impaired global and regional left ventricular function influence the prognosis in coronary artery disease with either medical treatment or coronary artery bypass surgery. Therefore, a noninvasive assessment of global and regional ventricular function should precede coronary angiography since it provides complementary information by predicting the functional response to improved myocardial perfusion after surgery. At present, radionuclide angiocardiography is probably the most promising technique for the noninvasive assessment of ventricular function.

First-Pass vs. Equilibrium Technique

Two basic approaches can be used for imaging of the heart cavities: (1) cumulative imaging with high temporal resolution (10–20 msec) using multiple gated acquisition after technetium-99m-labeled serum albumin or red blood cells have equilibrated in the blood pool, and (2) recording of the first pass of a ^{99m}Tc-pertechnetate bolus through the heart at a rate of 20–50 frames/sec.

The main advantage of the equilibrium technique is that it allows sequential measurements of global function to be obtained. For example, changes in ejection fraction during exercise can be measured with only one tracer injection. Frontal and left anterior oblique views can be recorded, but with all other projections there is a significant overlap of right and left heart chambers, which precludes regional analysis. With the first-pass technique, the right anterior oblique view can be used, as in invasive angiocardiography, for regional evaluation of left ventricular wall motion and ejection. The first-pass technique also allows compartmental analysis of right and left heart chamber function and lung function, such as evaluation of transit times, indicator dilution curves, and shunt ratios. Although repeated measurements require tracer reinjection, a scintillation camera system with a high count-rate capability (multicrystal type) permits several sequential injections to be performed.

Both techniques provide reliable information about global ventricular function, particularly the left ventricular ejection fraction [1, 2, 3]. When regional information is important, however, the first-pass technique is generally preferred.

Technical Problems

Technical problems involving image statistics, border definition, and motion analysis must be overcome for accurate assessment of ventricular performance. While these problems are clearly interrelated, they will be discussed separately.

The Image Statistics

Imaging of the left ventricle presents certain statistical difficulties because the radionuclide bolus is injected into a peripheral vein, distant from the left side of the heart. During the first transit, the bolus lengthens

Address reprint requests to. N. Schad, M.D., Strahlenabteilung, Städtisches Krankenhaus, D-8390 Passau, Federal Republic of Germany

and rapidly decreases in concentration. In addition, to resolve cardiac motion, count accumulation per frame is limited to 20–50 msec so that relatively low count densities result over the left ventricle.

Nevertheless, dynamic imaging of the left ventricle can be successfully performed if the bolus input into the right side of the heart is compact, the scintillation camera has high count capabilities (short dead times), and several cardiac cycles during the transit of the bolus through the left ventricle are summed to form a representative cycle [4]. Introduction of a compact bolus into the right side of the heart is routinely accomplished by the injection of a highly concentrated radionuclide bolus (18–20 mCi ^{99m}Tc-pertechnetate dissolved in 0.5 ml saline) into a large antecubital fossa vein or the external jugular vein. The vein is then flushed with 15 ml of saline at a flow rate of 6–8 ml/sec. The injection is timed so that the bolus arrives in the superior vena cava at ventricular diastole.

The flush-in technique keeps the bolus compact by reducing local diffusion of the radioactivity and by accelerating the venous flow to the superior vena cava. The injection is timed because diastolic arrival in the superior vena cava guarantees that the bolus will advance into the right atrium during the following systole, where it will accumulate since the tricuspid valve is closed during systole; systolic accumulation in the right atrium helps keep the bolus compact.

The multicrystal scintillation camera records up to 400,000 cps without saturation or the introduction of errors in the positioning of pulses, as it occurs with single crystal cameras at count rates over 80,000. Incorrect positioning, however, can introduce a certain degree of distortion and a general loss of spatial resolution. The sensitivity of multicrystal cameras, expressed as cps observed per 1 mCi bolus, is 10,000–16,000 cps in contrast to single-crystal cameras, which record only 4000 cps [5]. In fact, first-pass studies with multicrystal cameras, using the bolus-injection method outlined above, have produced count rates exceeding 200,000 cps in 240 consecutive examinations of our laboratory (Fig. 1).

Nevertheless, the activity distribution on a single short lasting frame produces a count density inadequate for satisfactory imaging. Therefore, six to nine cycles are summed to form a representative cycle. With the aid of the electrocardiogram and visual control, the first frames of the selected beats are individually chosen; all corresponding frames are subsequently added by a computer program. Precise determination of the initial frame of each cardiac phase avoids blurring of the information during the filling or emptying of cardiac chambers. Usually, only cycles on the wash-out side of left ventricular transit are added, guaranteeing adequate mixing and preventing the overlap of significant residual activity from the other chambers. The images of the representative cycle have higher count densities and, therefore, provide better statistical data. In addition, the resulting images of the representative cycle are linearly interpolated from a data matrix of 14×21 to one of 56×84 points.

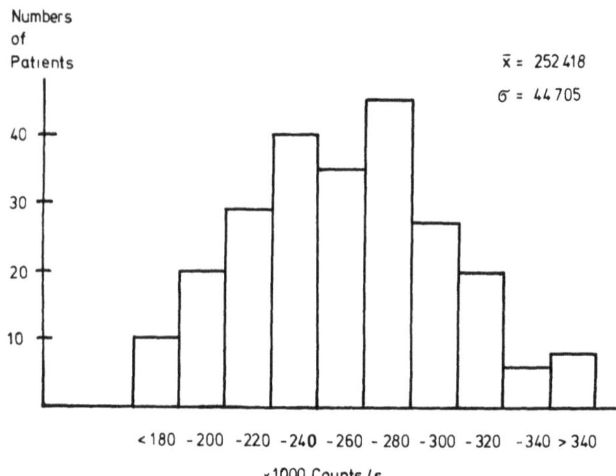

Fig. 1. During the first pass of the bolus through the heart, a maximum count rate of approximately 250,000 can be obtained by using a multicrystal camera and a compact bolus of 18–20 mCi ^{99m}Tc-pertechnetate. Note that in 96% of the 240 cases, a count rate greater than 180,000 cps was achieved.

Border Definition

Precise border definition on the representative cycle images is necessary for regional wall-motion analysis and for determination of heart size and ventricular volumes. Usually there is a gradual decrease in count density from the center of the heart chamber to the wall and the surrounding tissue or background. Therefore, detection of the heart border by simple visual control is frequently difficult, and assumption of a constant border background level is inaccurate, since the background varies from patient to patient. Thus, the first step in assessment of ventricular function is to define the left ventricular border and to eliminate from the image the background measured at that border [6].

Any border point has a statistical uncertainty corresponding to the square root of the count density at that point (Poisson statistics, standard deviation). Hence, the higher the count rate the relatively lower the percentage of statistical uncertainty (10% uncertainty with 100 counts vs. 5% uncertainty with 400 counts). Definition of a border point is possible when the change to the contiguous point is larger than the corresponding statistical uncertainty. Thus, the

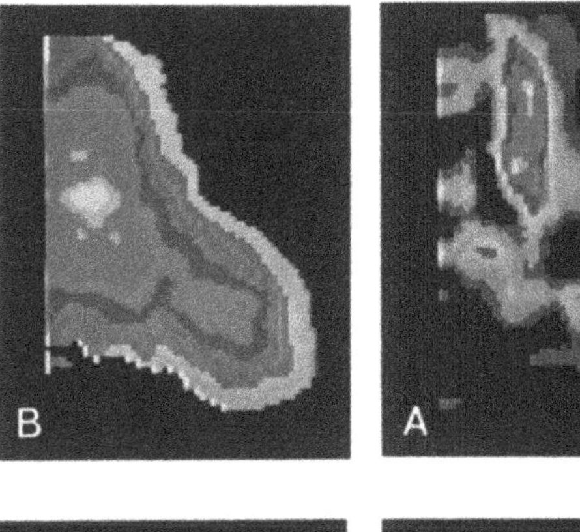

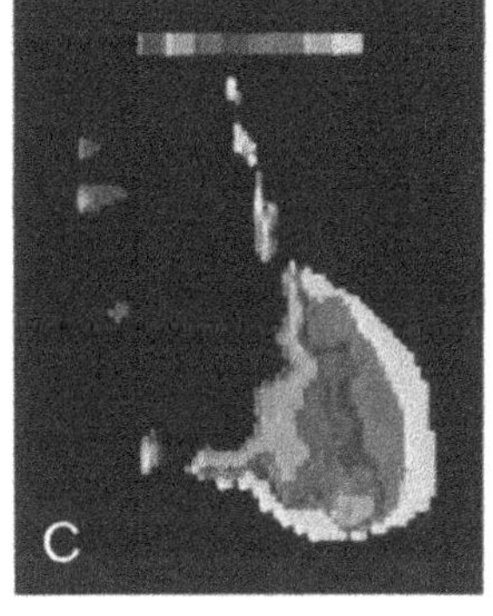

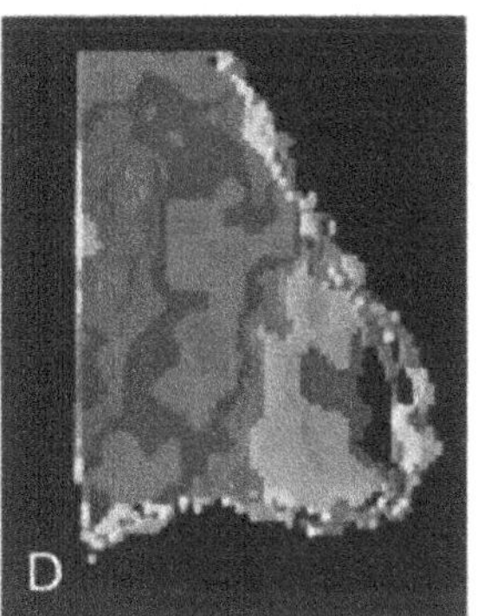

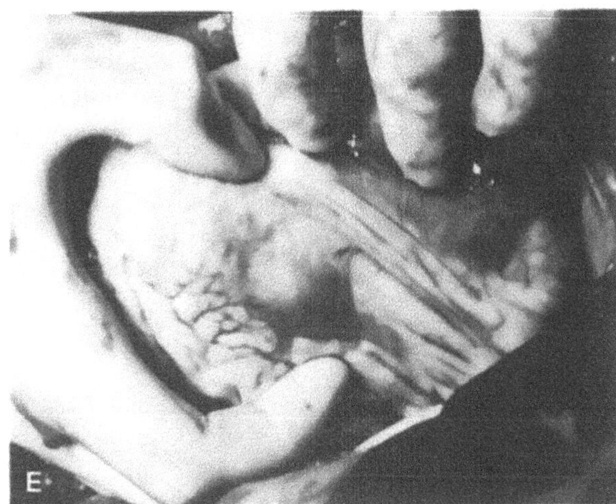

Fig. 2A–E. A 61-year-old patient with significant stenosis of the right coronary artery and first diagonal branch and 50% stenosis of the circumflex artery.
A Spatial gradient image derived from the end-diastolic left ventricular image of the representative cycle (right anterior oblique projection). Note the homogeneous increase in the gradient at the heart border.
B End-diastolic frame after border definition. From each border point a different background is eliminated, corresponding to the points of increase of the gradients.
C Regional ejection fraction image (10% incremental color scale). Hypokinesis is shown at the inferior wall (yellow band). Posterior to the apex, a small area of akinesis (shortening $<10\%$) and low regional ejection fraction (light blue and green) suggests a small aneurysm.
D Systolic mean transit time image. In contrast to **A–C**, this is derived by subtraction of a constant background; the heart is foreshortened at the apex. The shortest mean transit time is shown at the anterior wall where contraction is best (black and dark green), while at the inferior wall the transit time is prolonged (light blue). The small purple dot behind the apex points to long systolic persistence of activity in that area and suggests a small retroapical aneurysm.
E At coronary artery bypass surgery a small retroapical aneurysm of approximately fingertip size was found. (Photograph courtesy of Professor Klinner.)

steepness of change of count densities at the heart border becomes critical; in other words, a low background count and a high maximum count density over the heart chamber are of paramount importance [7]. Introduction of a compact tracer bolus into the right heart keeps the background count sufficiently low during left ventricular transit and count densities over the left ventricle sufficiently high to facilitate an accurate border determination.

A simple technique for detection of the ventricular border is to take a profile curve (count density distribution) through the center of the heart chamber, the two opposite walls, and the adjacent background. The border points are determined by taking the first or second derivative of the profile curve. The mean values at the two contiguous border points are considered as an approximation of the background of the chamber wall. Even in the same patient, however, the background levels vary around the left ventricular border and may also change during the cardiac cycle, so that another approach is required.

The principle of border definition can be expanded from one-dimensional profiles to the two-dimensional image. In two dimensions, the first derivative corresponds to the gradient of the two-dimensional density function of (x, y) or $f(i, k)$, $i=1 \ldots m$; $k=1 \ldots n$, which represents the image or matrix. This gradient is a vector; it contains information on the size and direction of changes in count density. For the determination of the heart border, only the size and not the direction of the gradient is important. Mathematically, the following function must be determined:

$$g(x, y)=\sqrt{\left(\frac{\partial f(x, y)}{\partial x}\right)^2+\left(\frac{\partial f(x, y)}{\partial y}\right)^2}.$$

This again can be represented by a matrix. The square of the function is the gradient image, $g^2(x, y)$ or $g^2(i, k)$. The maximum of the gradient image can be normalized to the maximum of the original image and both can be added together. The resulting image or the original gradient image is used for border definition.

On these gradient images – for example, those processed for the end-diastolic and end-systolic images (Fig. 2) – the densities at the heart border are in-

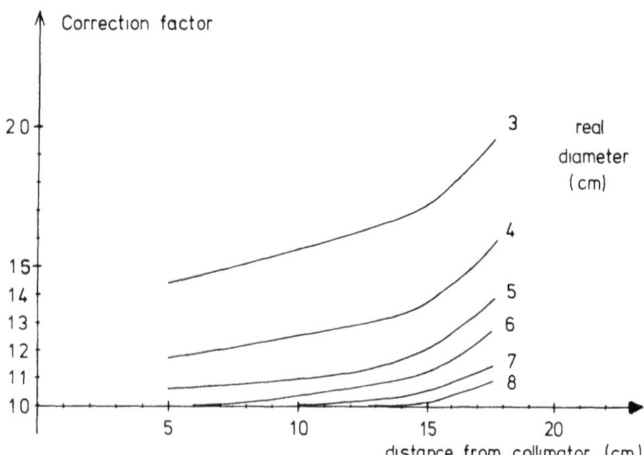

Fig. 3. Magnification factors for the diameters of images taken from circular dishes filled with ^{99m}Tc pertechnetate. The edges were defined by the same method used for left ventricular border definition in patients. For larger diameters (for example, the heart) magnification becomes small within a large range of distances (5–15 cm). (Reproduced from [6].)

creased and the background levels decreased, thus enhancing the contrast between the heart and its background. In addition, the background around the heart is more uniform on this image than on the original image, so that by setting a constant cut-off level and by forming a mask, the background around the original image can be easily eliminated. The main advantage of these images, however, lies in their improved definition of the heart border. This technique makes possible the accurate subtraction of the contiguous background from each border point. Segmental wall motion of the left ventricle measured by this technique has shown a high correspondence with segmental wall motion visualized by cineangiocardiography for normokinesis and asynergy (see below).

This technique also allows magnification factors to be calculated by measuring the images of small, circular ^{99m}Tc-pertechnetate-filled dishes of different diameters at various distances from the collimator. These magnification factors are needed for correction for actual volume measurements (Fig. 3).

Motion Analysis

The blurring effect of cardiac motion can be minimized by adapting the temporal resolution (frames per second) to the cardiac event and the information required. High temporal resolution, however, reduces count density so that it may become difficult to reach statistically valid diagnostic conclusions, particularly on regional image analysis. Thus, frame rate should be limited to the lowest acceptable level.

Can we detect motion of the heart border that is smaller than the static resolution of the system? Experimentally, 3 mm of motion can be resolved by moving the edge of a flood source 3 mm perpendicular to the edge and processing lines corresponding to the 50% count level (relative to the maximum density). Resolution depends on the count rate. If the maximum count density, Nmax, is only 50 instead of 500, fluctuations become too excessive to permit resolution of such small changes in the position of the edge.

In this way, one can define the minimum detectable motion of an edge as the "dynamic resolution," which follows the formula

$$\Delta x \approx \frac{1}{G}\sqrt{\frac{C}{N_{\max}}},$$

where G is the spatial gradient and C the relative density at a point x on the edge. The visible resolution, however, remains limited by the width of the matrix element (for example 0.27 cm). For practical purposes, aneurysms of fingertip size can be detected (Fig. 2).

Generally, regional changes between two sequential images can be demonstrated by subtracting the two images of end-diastole and end-systole. Subtraction, however, increases regional statistical noise disproportionally because the statistical fluctuation derives from the sum of both images but relates to their difference. Hence, within regions where changes are minimal, for example, where ventricular ejection is poor, statistical fluctuations are high on the subtraction image. Correspondingly, these regions are "noisy," poorly delineated, and difficult to separate from surrounding areas, and their function is not easily evaluated. However, it is precisely these regions that are the most important in regional diagnosis. Furthermore, by concentrating on only the two endpoints of the cardiac cycle one loses all information about what occurs throughout the entire period of ventricular contraction or relaxation [8].

To overcome these drawbacks, all regional changes during a total cardiac phase or part of that phase can be fitted (via least squares) to a given mathematical function so that an automatic smoothing of the data occurs. Single "temporally smoothed" images (for example, end-diastolic and end-systolic images) can then be used to process subtraction images, which contain fewer random fluctuations than the subtraction images obtained from the original images (linear or cosine fit).

Images that show the rate of linear decrease or increase in activity can also be processed; these images collect all information during a selected cardiac phase and reflect the average trend of density change during that phase for all matrix points (regional "temporal" gradients). This technique of temporal smoothing and averaging can be applied to count changes over the whole heart or over regions of the ventricle.

Noisy areas are automatically depressed by temporal smoothing, and the contrast between normal and abnormal regions is enhanced; areas with reduced or abnormal function are better delineated than on subtraction images, and the extent of malfunction becomes measurable. Therefore, trend images present a higher image quality and are diagnostically more reliable than subtraction images. Indeed, a high correlation has been found between areas of regional malfunction as shown on trend images and on cineangiocardiograms [8, 9].

Clinical Applications

Data on global and regional left and right ventricular function from first-pass radionuclide examinations are presented on time-activity curves computed over the ventricles and on the images of the left ventricular or right ventricular representative cycles, as well as on derived curves and images. In addition, global and regional information can be obtained at rest, after unloading the left ventricle by nitroglycerin administration, or while stressing it during exercise.

Information about global left ventricular function is prognostically important and may influence the decision of whether coronary artery bypass surgery or aneurysmectomy is indicated. Global assessments, however, include both regions with normal function and those with depressed function due to ischemia and/or scar formation. Hence, global parameters may to a certain degree mask regional disorders. Regional analysis, in addition, can be decisive in determining the treatment for patients with coronary artery disease.

Global Left Ventricular Function

Global information includes left ventricular ejection fraction, end-diastolic volume, and derived measurements, such as end-systolic volume, stroke volume, cardiac output, cardiac index, and systolic rate of ejection or ejection velocity. Measurement of global left ventricular ejection fraction by the first-pass technique correlates strongly ($r \approx 0.9$) with calculations from contrast angiocardiography [1,10–13]. It is a reliable parameter of left ventricular performance that can be directly computed from a time-activity curve of the representative cycle. The measurement is independent of assumptions about ventricular geometry that are introduced in computations of volume by the standard angiographic formula (i.e., that the ventricle can be approximated as a rotational ellipsoid). It also is not influenced by the projection used; the first-pass ejection fractions measured in the posteroanterior, right anterior oblique, and left anterior oblique projections, as well as in the left anterior oblique projection with a caudal tilt correlate well with the ejection fraction determinations derived from contrast angiography [10, 11, 14]. Furthermore, only small changes in ejection fraction were found on sequential measurements obtained over a four-day period ($4.4 \pm 3.6\%$) [15], so that the radionuclide determination of ejection fraction also represents a reproducible global parameter of left ventricular function. The same applies for the mean left ventricular ejection rate determined from the same representative cycle (slope of a fit to a weighted least squares straight line).

End-diastolic volume can be computed by definition of the left ventricular area on the end-diastolic image and the length of the major axis and by the use of the area-length method. Comparison between end-diastolic volumes determined by radionuclide techniques and by standard contrast biplane ventriculography showed a correlation coefficient of 0.89 in 33 patients [10]. In another study comparing ventriculography and radionuclide angiography, with both performed in the 30° right anterior oblique projection, the correlation coefficient of linear regression analysis was 0.93 [12]. From separate calculations of end-diastolic volume and ejection fraction, values can be derived for the end-systolic volume, stroke volume, cardiac output, and cardiac index. In 33 patients, comparison of cardiac output measured by an indocyanine green dye dilution curve and by radionuclide volumetric determination showed a correlation coefficient of 0.94 [16].

Regional Left Ventricular Function

Regional or segmental wall motion can be evaluated on first-pass radiocardiograms, particularly in the right anterior oblique projection. While the left anterior oblique view is reliable for evaluation of global left ventricular function (ejection fraction), the right anterior oblique view correlates better with contrast ventriculography for the detection and estimation of the severity of segmental wall motion abnormalities. Analysis of the predictive value of the left and right anterior oblique projections in asynergy showed a higher sensitivity and specificity for the right anterior oblique (sensitivity: left anterior oblique 0.62, right anterior oblique 0.74; specificity: left anterior oblique

Table 1. Correlation between radionuclide and contrast angiocardiography in the evaluation of segmental wall abnormalities

	Correlation between studies	
	Number of segments[a]	Percentage
Normal motion	129/142	91
Asynergy	61/68	90
Hypokinesis	38/43	88

[a] Total number=210 – Measurements of hemiaxis shortening

0.72, right anterior oblique 0.82) [17]. The right anterior oblique projection also showed a better correlation with contrast angiography than the left anterior oblique view in a grading of segmental involvement from 0 to 5+. Another study considering three left ventricular regions revealed agreement with the radiographic angiograms in 69 of 78 regions [18].

Obviously, the prerequisite for accurate regional wall motion analysis, as for volume determination, is the precise definition of the left ventricular border. By the use of spatial gradients for border detection (see above) and with measurements of wall motion in the right anterior oblique view, an average hemiaxis shortening for each of six segments per patient (210 segments in all) was computed in our laboratory on radionuclide and contrast angiograms of patients with coronary artery disease (Table 1). With normokinesis (hemiaxis shortening $\geq 30\%$) there was a correlation of 91% (129/142) between radionuclide and contrast studies; with motion disorders the correlation was 90% (61/68). Thus, detection of segmental asynergy in the right anterior oblique view was achieved with a sensitivity of 90% and a specificity of 91% with the first-pass technique. A correlation of 88% (38/43) was found with hypokinetic segments (hemiaxis shortening between 10 and 30%). Similar results were obtained in a study of another group with evaluation of wall motion by two independent observers [11].

The data confirm that by segmental wall motion analysis on first-pass right anterior oblique angiograms one can answer the clinically relevant question of whether there is normal or abnormal regional wall motion and whether hypokinesis is present with a high degree of certainty. Akinesis and dyskinesis, in our experience, are best evaluated on the functional images which express the average function throughout all of systole (i.e., the regional rate of decrease and increase and the mean transit-time image) because persistent akinesis or dyskinesis (of 300–400 ms) has greater clinical significance than does akinesis or dyskinesis that is limited to one or two images only (25–50 ms).

Important additional information about regional ejection is contributed by the derived functional images, such as regional distribution of stroke volume and ejection fractions (Fig. 2), rate of regional systolic decrease and increase, sinus fit images, and mean transit time images [4, 6, 8].

In our study of 210 segments, 142 displayed normal motion on contrast angiocardiography and 68 showed motion abnormalities. Nevertheless, 13 of the 142 with normal motion – all of which were at the base of the heart – were found to be hypokinetic (12) or akinetic (1) on radionuclide investigation. Considering wall motion separately, these segments would represent false-positive radionuclide angiographic segments. With all 13 segments, however, the adjacent zone of the left ventricular cavity showed depressed regional ejection on the functional images and a corresponding compromised vascular territory on the coronary angiogram. Therefore, the normokinetic contrast angiograms were considered falsely negative. The angiographic results can probably be explained as a consequence of the nitroglycerin the patients received during the procedure.

Seven of the 68 segments – all at the left ventricular apex – that showed motion disorders on contrast angiocardiography were found to be normokinetic by radionuclide studies. These segments represent false-negative radionuclide angiographic findings; the corresponding vascular territory was found to be compromised on the coronary angiogram for all segments. The adjacent regions of the left ventricular cavity however, showed a depressed regional function on the functional images; in all cases, data from the functional images thus, in effect, corrected for the false-negative regional wall motion findings. Similarily, of five of 43 hypokinetic segments shown on contrast angiograms, four apical segments were normokinetic on radionuclide angiograms and one posterobasal segment was akinetic. Again, all five segments showed reduced regional ejection in the adjacent zone, which served to correct for the false-negative information supplied by the normokinetic wall motion.

Thus, the information about regional wall motion and ejection obtained from first-pass radionuclide angiograms is both valuable and reliable. To increase the sensitivity and specificity, however, wall motion and ejection data from adjacent regions within the left ventricular cavity should always be evaluated together.

Right Ventricular Function

Global and regional information about right ventricular performance, which can also be noninvasively obtained from a first-pass study, allows the appropriate hemodynamic categorization of patients with pulmonary or left chamber disease and permits the evaluation of therapeutic interventions. In some instances when the right side of the heart is directly affected, analysis of global and regional right ventricular function can also provide valuable diagnostic information.

Global right ventricular ejection fractions have been measured in the left anterior oblique [19, 20] and anteroposterior projections [21] by averaging two to four beats during right ventricular bolus transit. Correlation with contrast angiocardiography was not feasible since contrast studies cannot accurately assess right ventricular volumes because of the irregular shape and trabeculated borders of the right ventricular cavity. Right ventricular ejection fraction measurements performed with peripheral vein injection correlated well, however, with those obtained with right atrial injection [19]. Mean normal values were $52\pm5\%$ [19], or 55% with a range of 45–65% (±2 SD) [21].

In patients with acute inferior myocardial infarctions examined on the first day after infarction, the right ventricular ejection fraction averaged $48\pm2\%$, which was significantly less than in patients with anterior infarctions ($56\pm2\%$, [21]). Right ventricular ejection fractions were lower in acute than in older infarcts, and were also significantly decreased in mitral stenosis [19] and cardiomyopathies [21].

In patients with clinically manifest cor pulmonale, the right ventricular ejection fraction was consistently and significantly decreased ($35\pm2\%$); several additional patients (4/19) with abnormal values developed cor pulmonale within one year after the study [21]. In chronic obstructive pulmonary disease, the right ventricular ejection fraction varied widely (19–71%); aminophyllin significantly increased the values. Also in cystic fibrosis, the range of ejection fraction values was large. Right ventricular performance in studies of ejection fraction was thus shown to correlate with the severity of ventilatory impairment, and to allow the early detection of right ventricular dysfunction before cor pulmonale developed.

Regionally, wall motion and ejection analysis is particularly helpful in the evaluation of patients with extended inferior infarctions involving both the posterobasal and diaphragmatic segments. All degrees of motion and ejection disorders known from the left ventricle have been observed at the inferior wall of the right ventricle. We have also found regional evaluation on functional right ventricular images to be of particular diagnostic value in cases with suspected tricuspid reflux in which systolic increase of activity could sometimes be demonstrated on the atrial side of the tricuspid valve, as well as in a patient with constrictive pericarditis who showed regional depressed wall motion and ejection in some of the calcified areas.

Exercise Studies

First-pass radionuclide angiocardiography during exercise can be used in screening patients for coronary artery disease. During excercise, potentially jeopardized myocardium will contract abnormally in patients with relatively normal function at rest. Graded bicycle exercise is frequently used, with measurements made when cardiac performance is maximally stressed. Patients who can only be exercised to angina and/or ischemic electrocardiographic changes or to symptom-limiting fatigue are examined at that level. The direction and magnitude of the left ventricular response is similar whether studies are performed with supine or upright exercise [13].

Global left ventricular function changes under stress as follows: In normal individuals, end-systolic volume decreases significantly, end-diastolic volume decreases slightly, and global ejection fraction increases during exercise (0.67 ± 0.08 to 0.8 ± 0.07) [10]. Also, in two other studies, normal individuals uniformly increased their ejection fractions with exercise by at least 10% ($66\pm2\%$ to $83\pm1\%$ and 0.65 ± 0.03 to 0.8 ± 0.03) [13, 22].

In a group of patients with significant one-vessel disease there was an equivalent increase in end-diastolic and stroke volume so that no change in ejection fraction resulted with exercise, whereas in a group of patients with multiple-vessel disease end-diastolic volume increased much more than stroke volume, so that the global ejection fraction decreased during stress (0.60 ± 0.14 to 0.53 ± 0.14) [10]. Most importantly, however, in both groups end-systolic volume increased in contrast to a control group of normal individuals. Successful revascularization reversed the pathologic response pattern [10, 23]: the ejection fraction response to exercise returned to normal in patients who became asymptomatic (0.64 ± 10 to 0.48 ± 0.09). Although some residual cardiac dilatation occurred in the asymptomatic group during exercise, the end-diastolic and end-systoliv volumes were less than before bypass surgery (Fig. 4).

A decrease in global ejection fraction during exercise in patients with significant coronary artery disease has been seen by other investigators: ($66\pm2\%$ to $57\pm2\%$) [13] and (0.57 ± 0.4 to 0.45 ± 0.03) [22]. While a 12-lead exercise electrocardiogram yielded false-negative studies in 36% (9/24) of patients with coronary artery disease, the radionuclide ejection fraction results were diagnostically accurate in all but

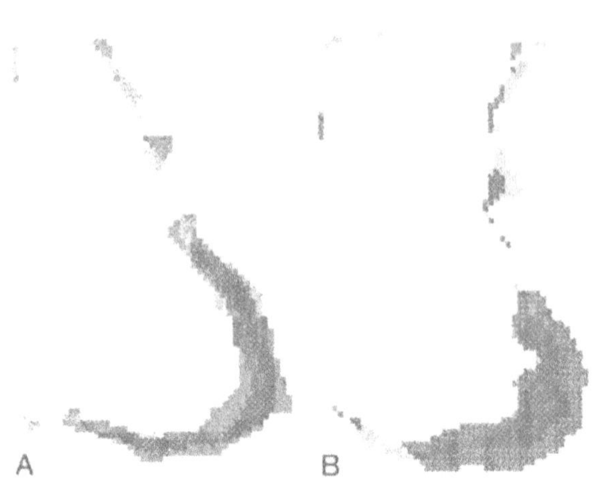

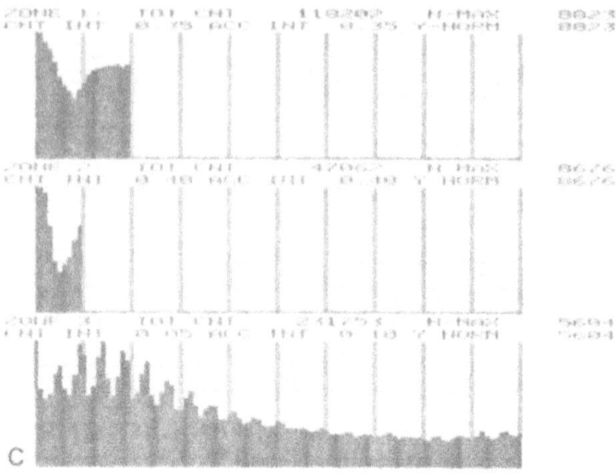

MEAN AGE 53 YEARS

	Rest	Exercise	P
Heart Rate (beats/min)	75±15	119±26	$<10^{-5}$
Cardiac Output (L/min)	5.7±1.5	11.3±4.3	$<10^{-5}$
Pulmonary Transit Time (sec)	7.7±1.8	5.4±1.7	$<10^{-5}$
Pulmonary Blood Volume (ml)	727±269	953±367	<.02

LEFT VENTRICULAR VOLUMES

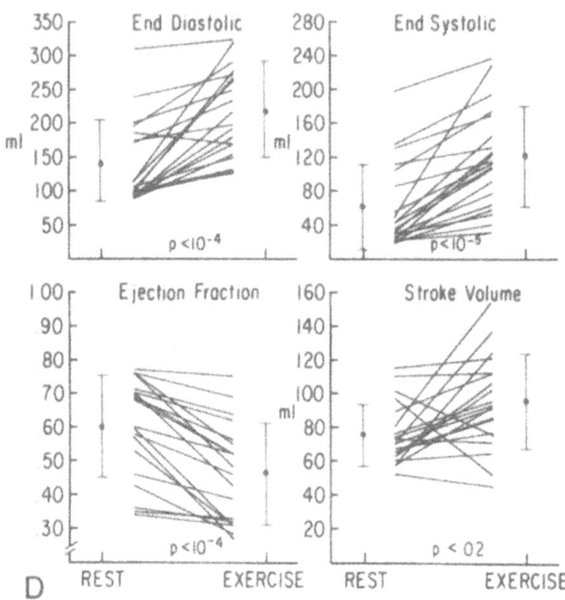

Fig. 4A–D. A 53-year-old patient with total occlusion of the left anterior descending artery after the origin of the first septal branch, retrograde filling of the left anterior descending artery by collateral flow, significant stenosis of the first diagonal branch, and 50% narrowing of the circumflex artery and marginal branch.
A Before surgery: wall motion trend image (systolic rate of decrease) at rest. Hypokinesis is shown at the inferior and anterobasal wall and the left ventricle is somewhat dilated. The patient was not stressed because of recurrent and increasing angina.
B Two months after coronary artery bypass surgery (three grafts): wall motion trend image after maximum exercise (heart rate, 124 beats/min). The left ventricle is smaller than it was before the surgery, and the strong, normal contraction in all segments suggests open grafts. A motion disorder of the posterobasal segment caused by prolapse of the mitral valve, which was apparent preoperatively, persists on this image.
C Global ejection fraction before (upper row) and after (middle row) surgery, left ventricular washout after surgery (lower row). The global ejection fraction rose from 53 to 69%. The left ventricular washout became normal after the surgery.
D Left ventricular response to exercise (end-diastolic and end-systolic volumes, ejection fraction, and stroke volume) in 20 patients with coronary artery disease involving more than one vessel. (Figure **D** courtesy of Dr. R.H. Jones.)

two patients with left anterior descending lesions of less than 70% and were also diagnostic in four patients with significant coronary artery disease on digoxin [24]. In patients in whom the ejection fraction does not change or decreases under stress, the resting ejection fraction is frequently normal, i.e., does not exclude significant coronary artery disease.

Regional left ventricular function at rest may also be normal or may already show circumscribed motion and ejection disorders. Normally during exercise, segmental wall motion and regional ejection increase uniformly. In areas supplied by stenosed coronary arteries, however, wall motion extent and regional ejection decrease. In patients with documented coronary artery disease who had either ischemic electrocardiographic changes and/or angina, the ejection fraction either fell or remained the same or even increased (52±4% to 58±4%) in contrast to patients with documented coronary artery disease who developed fatigue without detectable ischemia. New or exagerated regional wall motion abnormalities developed during exercise in both groups, including some patients in whom ejection fraction increased [13]. If only global information is considered, strong contraction in normal areas may mask depressed contractions in other areas, and no change or a slight increase in the ejection fraction may result. Therefore, regional wall motion and ejection analysis should always complement global evaluation. The exercise study usually enhances the regional contrast between the areas with normal and depressed function, and is thus helpful in defining the location and extent of the compromised vascular territory and in determining if disease of one or more vessels is present.

Exercise studies have been found particularly valuable in demonstrating the significance of a coronary stenosis and/or the adequacy of collateral perfusion [12]. Patients with coronary artery disease but insufficient collateralization were characterized by a significant decrease in ejection fraction and stroke volume in the presence of left ventricular dilatation at peak effort. Frequently (in 16 of 19 patients), new areas of wall motion dysfunction appeared at peak exercise. Some of the patients (4/11) with visualized collaterals to all major cornary arteries also showed new areas of wall motion dysfunction and a decrease in ejection fraction at peak effort, suggesting functionally inadequate collateralization.

Exercise functional images are particularly helpful for following patients after revascularization procedures since they can demonstrate the adequacy of bypass flow to the originally compromised territories. Segmental wall motion abnormalities that occur during exercise may disappear after successful bypass surgery, and a global left ventricular decrease in wall excursion during exercise may markedly improve (Fig. 4).

Exercise studies can also be helpful in the detection of latent heart failure before it becomes clinically manifest in patients with valvular heart disease, (e.g., aortic insufficiency) [23]. Patients who had decreased ejection fraction with exercise before aortic and mitral valve replacement were found to represent a higher operative risk than patients who had an increased ejection fraction [23].

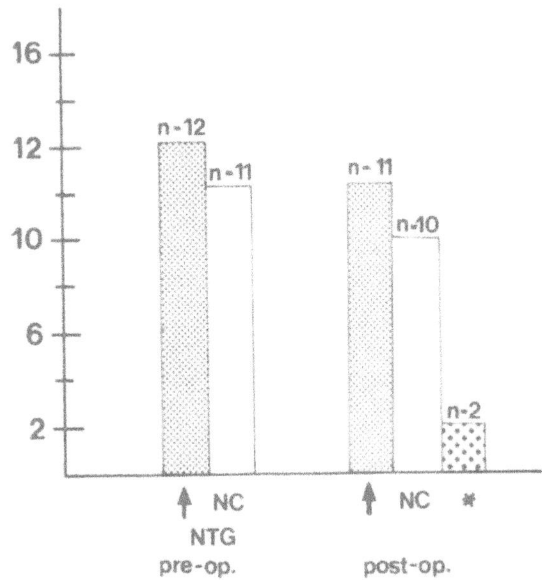

Fig. 5. Predictive value of nitroglycerin intervention first-pass studies for akinetic segments. Of 23 akinetic segments, 12 improved after nitroglycerin; 11 of the 12 also improved after surgery. The improvement of one akinetic segment after surgery was not predicted by the results of the nitroglycerin study. (Figure courtesy of Dr. C.K. Hellman.)

Nitroglycerin Administration

Screening for reversible as opposed to nonreversible depression of left ventricular function has rested on two tests performed during invasive cardiac catheterization and contrast ventriculography: post-extra systolic potentiation and nitroglycerin potentiation. The latter, however, can be noninvasively performed using first-pass right anterior oblique radionuclide angiocardiography; global ejection fraction and regional wall motion and ejection can be examined before and after nitroglycerin administration. The examination allows one to determine whether function in severely hypokinetic or akinetic regions improves after nitroglycerin or remains unchanged, thereby suggesting extensive scar formation.

In 44 patients with documented myocardial infarction examined before and after sublingual nitroglycerin administration, we observed an average increase in global ejection fraction of 6%. In two other recent studies the increase was 6% [25] and 7% [12]. In the same patients the average resting ejection fraction rose from 40 to 46% with nitroglycerin, while after bypass surgery it rose from 32 to 40%. The preoperative ejection fraction after nitroglycerin and the postoperative ejection fraction after bypass surgery showed an acceptable correlation [12].

When ejection fraction, ejection velocity, and end-diastolic volumes at rest, after nitroglycerin, and postoperatively were compared [25], a significant difference was found between the resting and nitroglycerin data, but no significant difference between the nitroglycerin and postoperative data. Regional wall motion analysis on a total of 120 segments showed similar changes: no improvement of dyskinetic segments

Table 2. Regional wall motion before and after nitroglycerin administration

Wall motion	Number of segments[a]		
	Before nitroglycerin	After nitroglycerin	Overall change
Normokinetic	81	122 (+50.6%)	+18.6%
Hypokinetic	102	80 (−21.6%)	−10.0%
Akinetic	32	13 (−60.0%)	− 8.6%
Dyskinetic	5	5	None

[a] Total number=220 – Measurements of hemiaxis shortening

(8/120) after either nitroglycerin or bypass surgery and improvement of approximately half of hypokinetic and akinetic segments following nitroglycerin and surgery (Fig. 5); only a small number (9/120) showed improvement after surgery that was not predicted by the results with nitroglycerin [14]. The studies showed a sensitivity of 81% and a specificity of 81% in predicting potential wall motion improvement after revascularization. By the use of a newly designed bilateral collimator giving both fixed 30° right anterior oblique and 30° left anterior oblique views simultaneously, an identical sensitivity of 81% was found, but specificity was increased to 97% [14].

Regional wall motion was evaluated in our laboratory in 44 patients with documented myocardial infarctions. Average hemiaxis shortening was measured in five left ventricular segments (anterobasal, anterior, apical, diaphragmatic and posterobasal) in each patient (220 segments in all). After nitroglycerin administration, the number of segments with normal motion (>25% shortening) increased 51%, the number with hypokinesis (11–25% shortening) decreased 22%, and the number with akinesis decreased 60% (Table 2). All infarcted segments (44) showed motion disorders; 70% of the hypokinetic and 67% of the akinetic segments improved after nitroglycerin, but no response was observed in the four dyskinetic segments (Fig. 6). Fifty-four percent of 59 adjacent segments showed a motion disorder; three-fourths of these segments improved after nitroglycerin. No difference was observed in the response pattern of anterior and inferior infarcts (Fig. 7).

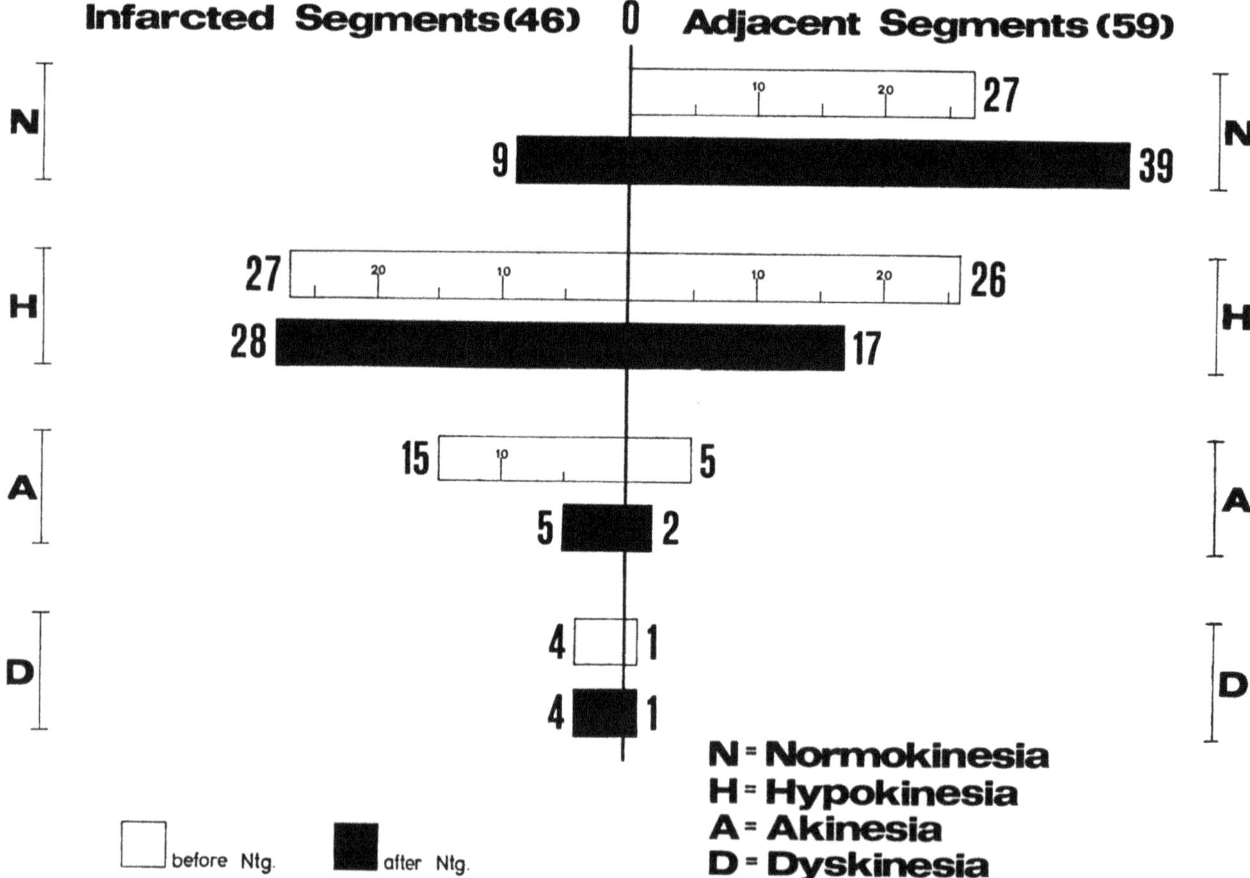

Fig. 6. Nitroglycerin response in infarcted (left) and adjacent (right) left ventricular segments. No response was shown in the dyskinetic regions. Thirteen (67%) of the akinetic segments became hypokinetic. The number of segments displaying normal motion increased by 21; more of the segments adjacent to infarcted regions showed normalization of motion than did the infarcted segments.

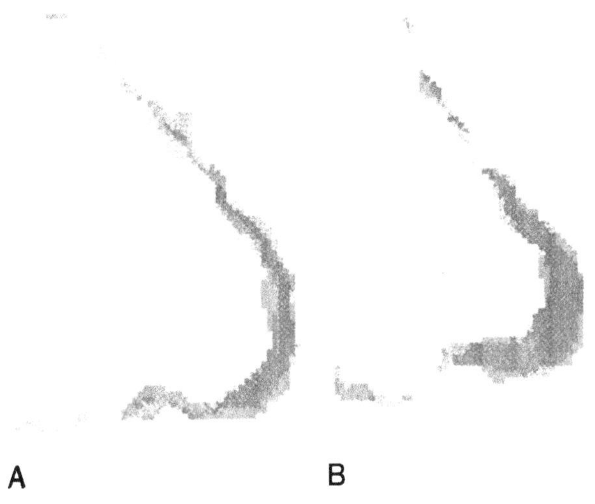

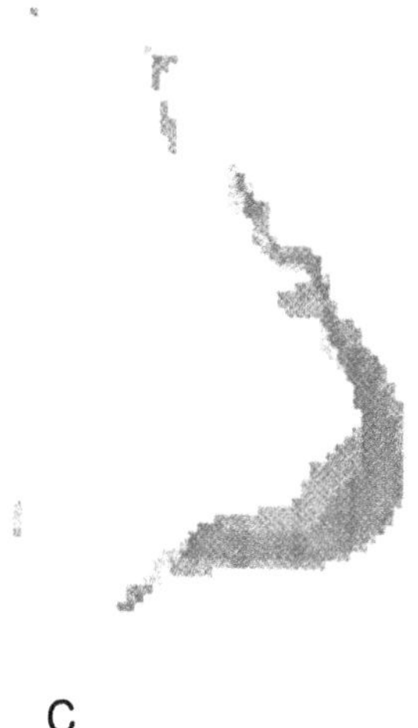

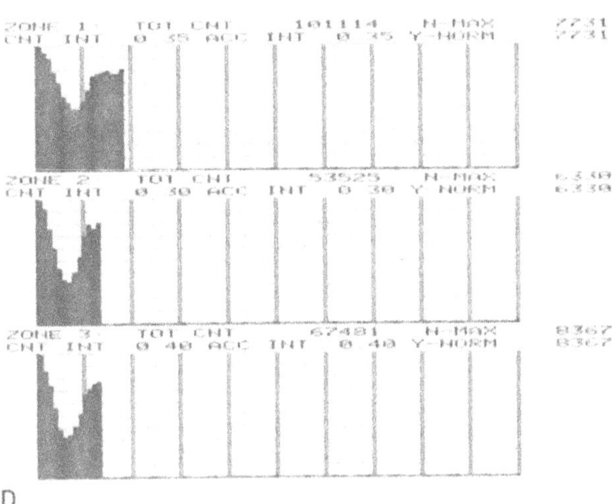

Fig. 7 A–D. A 41-year-old patient with significant stenosis of the left anterior descending artery after the origin of a severely narrowed first diagonal branch as well as significant stenosis of the circumflex artery.
A Before surgery: wall motion trend image (systolic rate of decrease) at rest. The left ventricle is dilated and hypokinetic at its inferior and anterobasal wall. The patient was not stressed because of increasing angina.
B Eighteen days after coronary artery bypass surgery (two grafts): wall motion trend image before nitroglycerin administration. The left ventricle is smaller. Improved and normalized motion, which is shown in all segments, particularly at the inferior, apical and supra-apical wall, suggests open grafts.
C Twelve minutes after nitroglycerin administration. Further improvement is evident at the inferior wall and at the apex. The somewhat reduced motion at the anterobasal wall is probably due to the severely narrowed first diagonal branch, which could not be grafted.
D Global ejection fraction before (upper) and after surgery (middle) and after nitroglycerin (lower). The global ejection fraction rose from 52% before surgery to 66% after surgery and to 69% after nitroglycerin.

References

1. Ashburn, W.L., Schelbert, H.R., Verba, J.W.: Left ventricular ejection fraction: A review of several radionuclide angiographic approaches using the scintillation camera. Principles of Cardiovascular Nuclear Medicine, edited by B.L. Holman, E.H. Sonnenblick, M. Lesch. New York, Grune & Stratton, 1978, pp. 171–188
2. Pierson, R.N.: Application of ventricular function in the acute care environment: First transit and gated studies. Symposium on Nuclear Cardiology: Principles and Applications. Milwaukee, October 1978
3. Strauss, H.W., Pitt, B.: Gated cardiac blood-pool scan: Use in patients with coronary heart disease. Principles of Cardiovascular Nuclear Medicine, edited by B.L. Holman, E.H. Sonnenblick, M. Lesch. New York, Grune & Stratton, 1978, pp. 161–170
4. Schad, N.: Nontraumatic assessment of left ventricular wall motion and regional stroke volume after myocardial infarction. J. Nucl. Med. 18:333–341, 1977
5. MacIntyre, W.J.: Imaging devices and computers in nuclear cardiology. Symposium on nuclear cardiology: Principles and applications. Milwaukee, October 1978
6. Nickel, O., Schad, N.: Image analysis of the heart action recorded with a high speed multicrystal gamma camera. Med. Progr. Technol. 5:1–7, 1978
7. Budinger, T.F., Rollo, F.D.: Physics and instrumentation. Principles of Cardiovascular Nuclear Medicine, edited by B.L. Holman, E.H. Sonnenblick, M. Lesch. New York, Grune & Stratton 1978, pp. 17–51
8. Schad, N., Nickel, O.: Radionuclide angiography in coronary heart disease: Where do we stand? Cardiovasc. Radiol. 1:27–35, 1978
9. Ramos, M., Rösler, H., Neolpp, U., Salzmann, C., Fritschy, P.: Trend scintigrams in the work-up of cardiac patients (abstract). World Federation of Nuclear Medicine and Biology: Second International Congress, Washington, D.C., Sept. 17–21, 1978, p. 4
10. Jones, R.H., Rerych, S.K., Newman, G.E., Scholz, P.M., Howe, W.R., Oldham, H.N., Goodrich, J.K., Sabiston, D.C.: Noninvasive radionuclide procedures for diagnosis and management of myocardial ischemia. World J. Surg. 2:811–824, 1978
11. Schmid, D.H.: First pass technique. Symposium on Nuclear Cardiology. Regensburg, September 1978
12. Hellman, C.K.: Dynamic evaluation of ventricular function. Symposium on Nuclear Cardiology: Principles and Applications. Milwaukee, October 1978

13. Berger, H., Reduto, L., Johnstone, D., Sands, M., Borkowski, H., Langou, R., Cohen, L., Gottschalk, A., Zaret, B.: Radionuclide assessment of global and regional left ventricular function during graded bicycle exercise in coronary artery disease (abstract). World Federation of Nuclear Medicine and Biology: Second International Congress, Washington, D.C., Sept. 17–21, 1978, p. 2
14. Tow, D.E., Parisi, A.F., Folland, E., Sasahara, A.A., Dilts, C.A.: Quantative radionuclide (RN) assessment of left ventricular function (LVF): Precision and correlation with contrast angiography (abstract). World Federation of Nuclear Medicine and Biology: Second International Congress, Washington, D.C. Sept. 17–21, 1978, p. 99
15. Marshall, R.C., Berger, H.J., Reduto, L.A., Gottschalk, A., Zaret, B.L.: Variability in sequential measure of left ventricular performance assessed with radionuclide angiocardiography. Am. J. Cardiol. 41: 531–536, 1978
16. Rerych, S.K., Scholz, P.M., Newman, G.E., Sabiston, D.C., Jones, R.H.: Cardiac function at rest and during exercise in normals and in patients with coronary heart disease: Evaluation by radionuclide angiocardiography. Ann. Surg. 187: 449, 1978
17. Ally, K., Patterson, R., Horowitz, S.F., Pichard, A., Herman, M.V., Gorlin, R., Goldsmith, S.J.: Relative merit of RAO and LAO radionuclide angiocardiography in the detection of left ventricular regional wall motion abnormalities (abstract). World Federation of Nuclear Medicine and Biology: Second International Congress, Washington, D.C., Sept. 17–21, 1978, p. 139
18. Shields, R.A., Walton, S., Wrigley, C., Rowlands, D.J., Testa, H.J.: Left-ventricular wall motion by first passage radionuclide angiocardiography (abstract). World Federation of Nuclear Medicine and Biology: Second International Congress, Washington, D.C., Sept. 17–21, 1978, p. 95
19. Suzuki, Y., Kanemoto, N.: Noninvasive measurement of right ventricular ejection fraction with radionuclide angiocardiography (abstract). World Federation of Nuclear Medicine and Biology: Second International Congress, Washington, D.C., Sept. 17–21, 1978, p. 52
20. Zita, G., Zwick, H., Kubicek, F., Koriska, K., Schultschik, R.: Haemodynamic findings in pulmonary hypertension (abstract). World Federation of Nuclear Medicine and Biology: Second International Congress, Washington, D.C., Sept. 17–21, 1978, p. 53
21. Berger, H., Zaret, B.: Quantitative assessment of right ventricular performance by first-pass radionuclide angiocardiography: Clinical applications in cardiopulmonary disease (abstract). World Federation of Nuclear Medicine and Biology: Second International Congress, Washington, D.C., Sept. 17–21, 1978, p. 53
22. Jengo, J.A., Uszler, J.M., Freeman, R., Oren, V., Mena, I.: Upright exercise stress first pass radionuclide detection of coronary artery disease (abstract). World Federation of Nuclear Medicine and Biology: Second International Congress, Washington, D.C., Sept. 17–21, 1978, p. 95
23. Jones, R.H., Newman, G.E., Rerych, S.K., Scholz, P.M., Upton, M.T., Sabiston, D.C.: Rest and exercise radionuclide angiocardiography in surgical patients (abstract). World Federation of Nuclear Medicine and Biology: Second International Congress, Washington, D.C., Sept. 17–21, 1978, p. 95
24. Lumina, F., Germon, P., Maranhoe, V., Cha, S., Gooch, A., Goldberg, H.: Comparison of radionuclide angiography with stress testing in the diagnosis of CAD (abstract). World Federation of Nuclear Medicine and Biology: Second International Congress, Washington, D.C., Sept. 17–21, 1978, p. 153
25 Kremers, S., Kight, J., Heck, L., Van Hove, E.: Value of nitroglycerine radionuclide angiocardiography in preoperative evaluation of patients with coronary artery disease (abstract). World Federation of Nuclear Medicine and Biology: Second International Congress, Washington, D.C., Sept. 17–21, 1978, p. 23

Equilibrium (Gated) Radionuclide Ventriculography

W.E. Adam,[1] A. Tarkowska,[2] F. Bitter,[1] M. Stauch,[3] and H. Geffers[1]

[1] Department of Radiology III (Nuclear Medicine), Ulm University, Ulm, FRG
[2] Department of Nuclear Medicine, Medical School, Lublin, Poland
[3] Section of Cardiology, Ulm University, Ulm, FRG

Equilibrium (gated) radionuclide ventriculography is based on the fact that the heart is a periodically contracting organ. The amount of radioactivity in the heart is proportional to the amount of blood in its cavities, provided there is homogeneous distribution in the blood pool. Thus, the precordial count rate changes reflect the cyclic volume changes of the heart. Because the precordial count rate is too low for a reliable determination of a beat-by-beat time-volume curve, Hoffmann and Kleine applied a gating procedure, using the R-wave of the electrocardiograph (ECG) and a multichannel analyzer [24] to synchronize and sum hundreds of heart cycles. This resulted in a representative cardiac cycle and a well-delineated time-activity curve, which is analogous to a time-volume curve. Since the left and right ventricles could not be differentiated by this technique, and an additional x-ray investigation was required for their delineation, Adam et al. [1, 4] and Bitter et al. [9] applied the gating procedure to a camera computer system. Representative time-activity (time-volume) curves of the left and right ventricle were obtained using an electronic cursor to isolate the ventricles.

Finally, a set of regional time-activity curves was obtained, each one presenting the cardiac cycle of one small region corresponding to the resolution of the camera computer system [2, 8, 16] (Fig. 1). This technique allows the state of any point of the heart at any moment of the cardiac cycle to be defined. To bring that vast amount of data into a manageable form, European investigators employed the "functional imaging" or "parametric scan" procedure developed in the United States by MacIntyre and Loken [31, 35]. In this method, the various parameters of the regional curves are assessed separately (Fig. 2). For example the computer can plot all regions with a greater than 30% reduction in amplitude in black, thus clearly outlining the hypokinetic regions. In the next parametric scan all regional curves may be analyzed in terms of their respective synchronous contraction, with all regions with a delayed contraction of more than, for example, 20% being plotted in black so that dyskinetic regions would be outlined. By this method, a set of parametric scans is constructed that allows detailed analysis of heart wall motion.

In contrast to the various European groups [3, 5, 8, 12, 13, 14, 16, 18, 26–29, 32, 33], research groups in the United States have applied the gated-blood-pool method to obtain images in various phases of the heart cycle [21, 37–42, 44, 45, 52–54]. Using this technique Zaret et al. detected regional ventricular dysfunction in man and measured the left ventricular ejection fraction [55, 57]. These authors started with imaging at two points in the cardiac cycle (end-systole and end-diastole). Later multiple gated images over the whole cycle length were obtained (Figs. 3 and 4). These data were combined and displayed in real time as an endless loop. These radionuclide cineventriculograms allowed the detection of wall motion abnormalities by simple inspection, though they did not utilize all the information contained in the investigations. The movie mode is similar to contrast cineventriculography, though the radionuclide method has the advantage of being noninvasive and the disadvantage of providing limited spatial resolution. The cine mode is only a qualitative method, in contrast to the parametric scan mode, which provides quantitative information.

An important new application of the gated blood pool procedure was introduced by Borer et al. [10, 11] and Green and Borer [19], who performed it during stress, thereby confirming and localizing coronary artery disease by the detection of wall motion abnorma-

Supported by the Bundesministerium für Forschung und Technologie, Bonn, FRG

Address reprint requests to: Prof. Dr. W.E. Adam, Department of Radiology III (Nuclear Medicine), Ulm University, Steinhövelstraße 9, D-7900 Ulm, Federal Republic of Germany

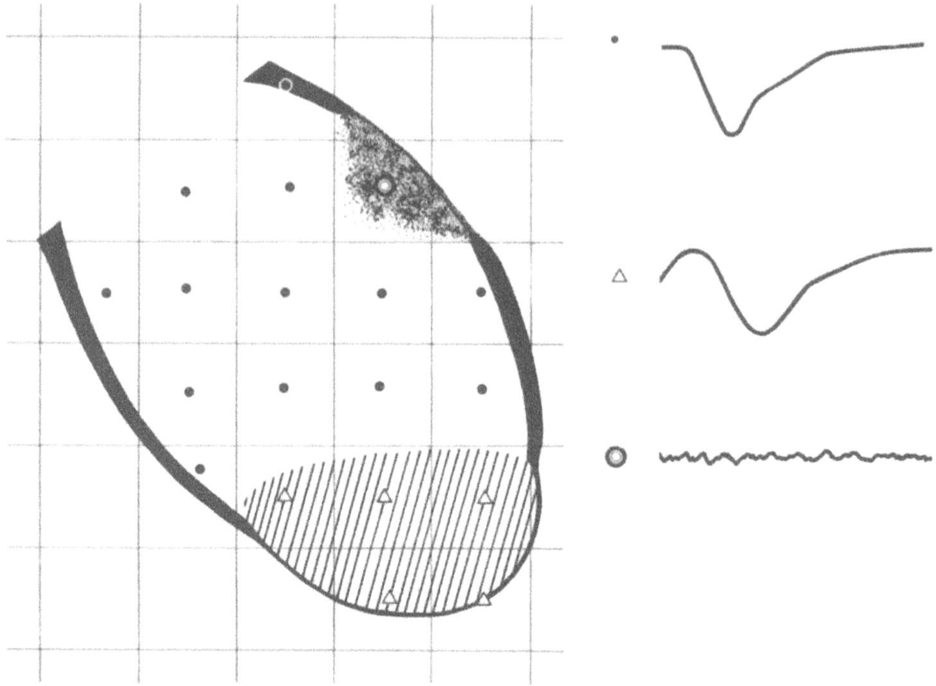

Fig. 1. Detailed analysis of gated blood pool data utilizes the region of interest technique. The result equals that of a set of small detectors, arranged in matrix form, with each detector observing one small region of the heart, and registering a time-activity curve that corresponds to the time-volume curve of the area. Typical time-activity curves are illustrated for normokinetic regions *(upper right)*, dyskinetic regions with phase shifting and delayed systole *(middle right)*, and akinetic regions with no systematic behaviour except statistical noise *(lower right)*. For the left ventricular area a set of 30–350 curves are produced, depending on the ventricular size. This set of regional curves is the basis for further analysis.

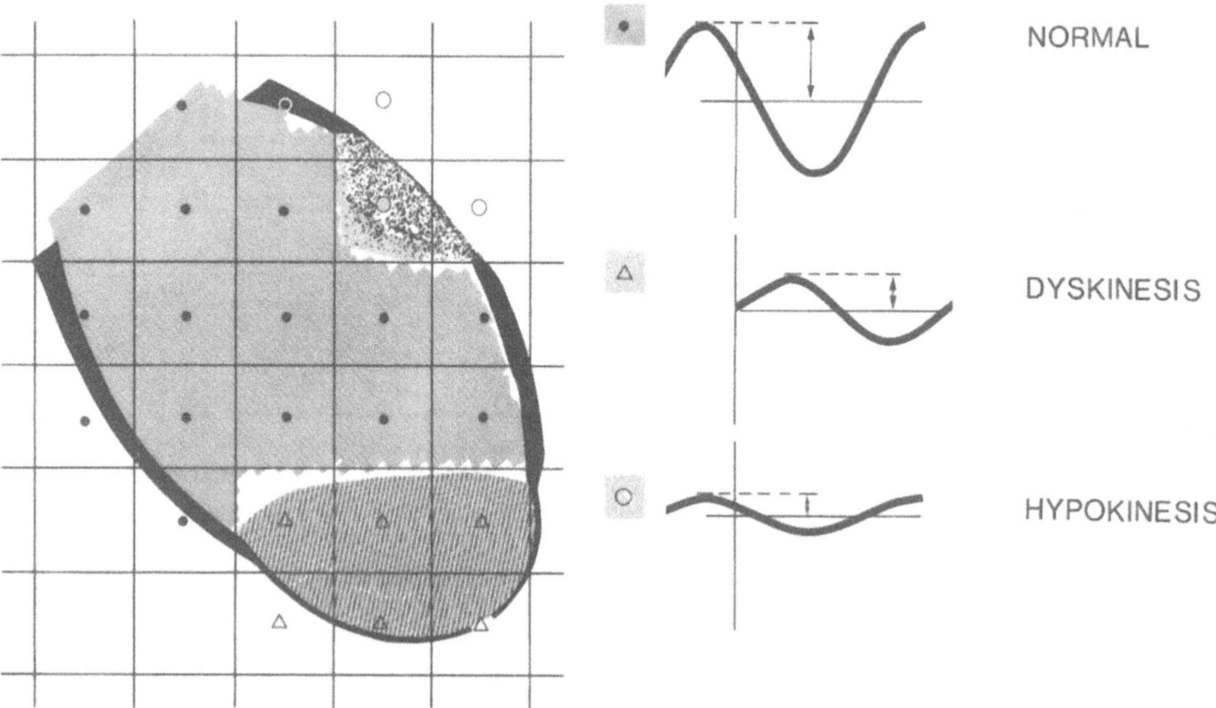

Fig. 2. Example of a parametric scan. The amplitude of the first Fourier element of the regional curves is utilized as the parameter. The distribution of the amplitudes is plotted in gray scale. Hypokinetic areas and dyskinetic regions with small amplitudes are visualized.

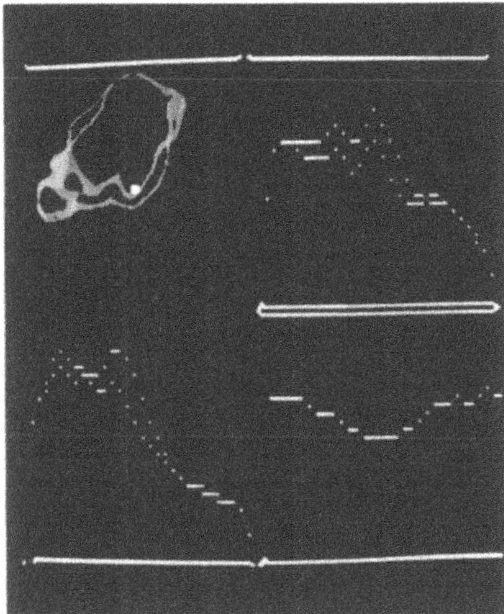

Fig. 3. The cineventriculogram (qualitative evaluation). The n phasic frames are displayed in an endless loop, resulting in a cinematic effect (the "beating heart" on the *top left*). The regional time-activity (time-volume) curve (*lower right*) corresponds to the apical left ventricular region of the small (white) marker. On the *top right*, the radioactivity profile of the line and, on the *lower left*, the profile of the column crossing the marker are shown. Both profiles indicate cyclic wall motions perpendicular to the plane. The profiles are presented in end-diastole and end-systole. The marker can be placed into various regions, as desired, to indicate regional motility.

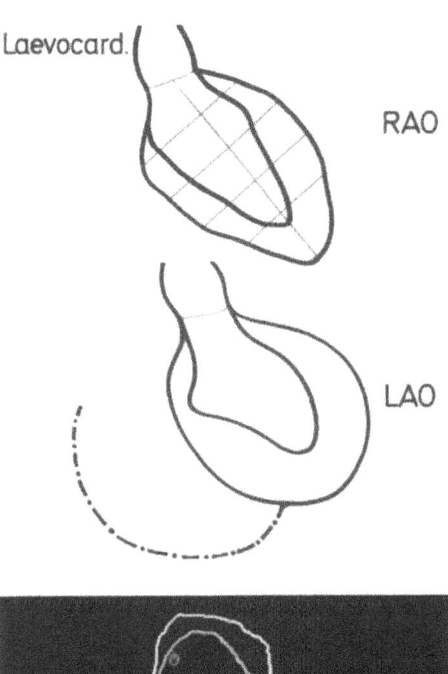

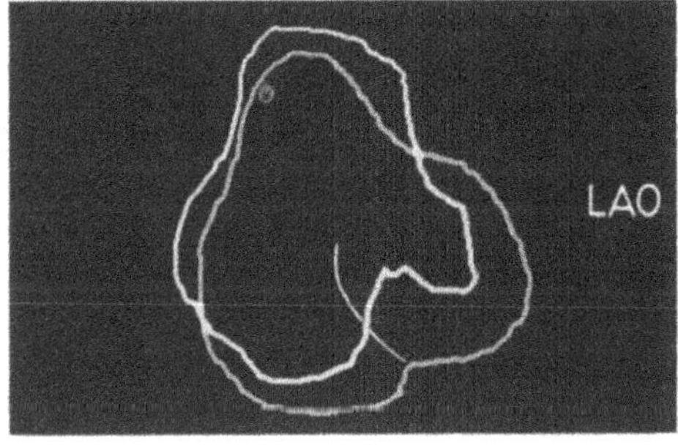

Fig. 4. Biplane ventriculography *(upper and center picture)* and radionuclide ventriculography *(lower picture)*. For imaging of the left ventricle without overlapping, the left anterior oblique position is obligatory in radionuclide ventriculography. Comparison of end-diastolic and end-systolic contours provides information concerning regional and global myocardial wall motion.

lities in the areas supplied by the obstructed arteries. The "nuclear stethoscope," a low-cost single-detector device, was developed by Wagner et al. [56] to allow imaging of the left ventricular time-volume curve and calculate the ejection fraction. This simple mobile device may become an important tool on intensive care wards [7].

Technique and Data Acquisition

For gated ventriculography, 15–20 mCi of technetium-99m labeled human serum albumin or red blood cells are injected intravenously. After homogeneous tracer distribution in the blood pool, the camera detector is placed over the heart perpendicular to the septum, usually at a 30° left anterior oblique angle. The right and left sides of the heart can then be differentiated.

Data acquisition requires about four to 15 minutes and provides from 16 to 64 frames of one heart cycle, each describing one short phase of the cycle (about 5–50 msec). For statistical reasons, each frame should be built up of at least 400,000 counts if regional details are to be quantitated; thus, the whole investigation consists of 6.4 to 25.6 million counts. Because the precordial count rate is about 30,000 cps, the total imaging time ranges from four to 15 minutes.

Since the time-activity curve is made up of hundreds of cardiac cycles, exact synchronization is required. Synchronization deteriorates toward the end of the cycle and with the distance from the trigger signal (R-wave). For this reason some groups prefer forward and backward gating after the data is acquired in list mode, which ensures better synchronization of the last frames of the heart cycle [19–21, 34]. Data acquisition can be performed in synchronized frame mode or in list mode. List mode is more cumbersome and time-consuming, storing all the original counts and the ECG information on magnetic tape or a large disc. Reformation into a gated study is done during replay from tape or disc, allowing selection of cycles of specific length. We prefer the synchronized frame mode, which builds up the set of requested frames in the core memory during the data acquisition. In this mode some corrections must be performed to ensure accuracy: (1) determination of the mean cycle length preceding the start of the data acquisition; (2) online presentation of cycle length, variations, and trends during the investigation; and (3) elimination of extra-systolic heart beats. All these functions are performed by the computer.

Employing a 30° left anterior oblique projection causes overlapping of the anterior and posterior myocardial walls; to differentiate the walls, a second investigation is necessary in a 60° left anterior oblique projection. The repetition of the investigation causes no difficulties as long as sufficient activity remains in the blood pool. Follow-up investigations under varying conditions are also possible. Repetition under stress conditions as performed with a bicycle ergometer in the supine position can reveal regional motility abnormalities in patients with coronary artery disease and limited coronary reserve. Synchronization can present certain problems in stress investigations; however, we have found that the heart rate remains surprisingly constant when the full stress load has been reached, so that good data can still be obtained in synchronized frame mode.

Methods of Data Analysis

Qualitative Evaluation: Radionuclide Cineventriculography

The rapid sequential display of the frames of the radionuclide ventriculogram in an endless loop produces a cinematic effect; the heart appears to beat. Akinetic and dyskinetic regions of the heart wall are visualized and correspond to wall motion abnormalities demonstrated on the contrast cineangiocardiogram. Scars are usually visible only when they are on the rim of the ventricle image (Fig. 5), and gray-scale changes within the contour sometimes escape detection. For this reason, a marker can be placed into each region of the heart (Fig. 3). The corresponding regional time-activity (time-volume) curve is visualized, and the column and line of the scan matrix crossing in the marker point are displayed. These procedures show heart wall motion in a direction perpendicular to the observer and provide a three-dimensional image which allows visualization of scars in the center of the ventricle.

Quantitative Evaluation

The set of n frames of one average cardiac cycle can also be used to evaluate left ventricular global and regional function.

Assessment of Left Ventricular Global Function

The precordial cyclic count-rate changes correspond to volume changes of the heart if the left ventricular contour is correctly drawn and accurate background corrections are performed. The most critical element in background subtraction is usually the accurate outlining of the heart contour. Applying a Fourier anal-

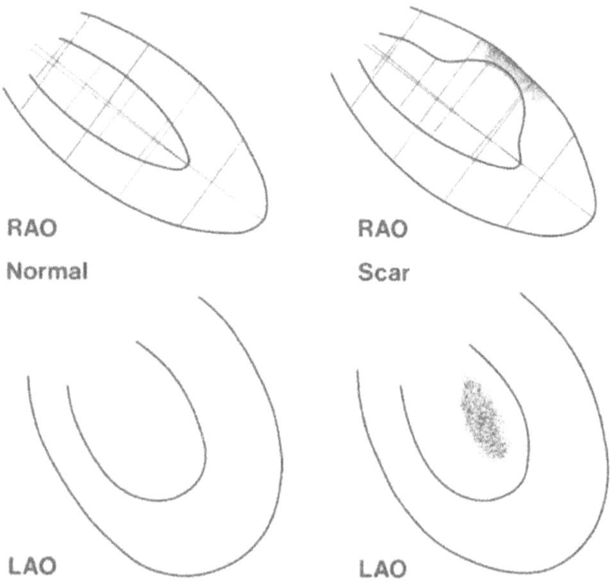

RAO Normal

RAO Scar

LAO

LAO

Fig. 5. Contour plotting has disadvantages. While scars are clearly visible in regions tangential to the detector *(upper right)*, they may escape detection when they are in the center of the ventricle *(lower right)*.

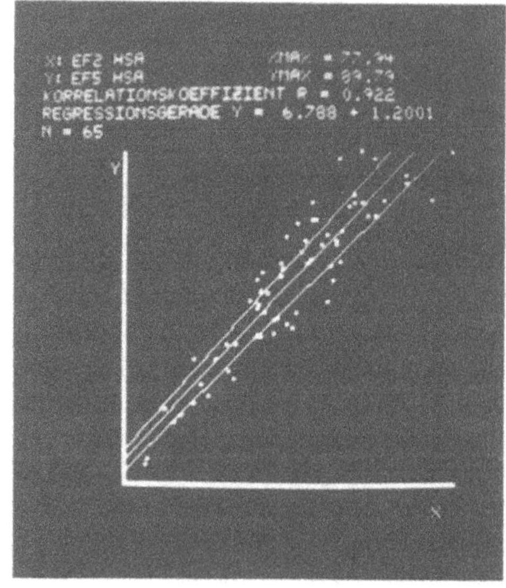

Fig. 6. Ejection fraction assessment. The "horizontal plane" (x) subtraction underestimates the ejection fraction. The background subtraction by an "inclined plane" (y) yields higher values (+20%), which are in agreement with clinical results.

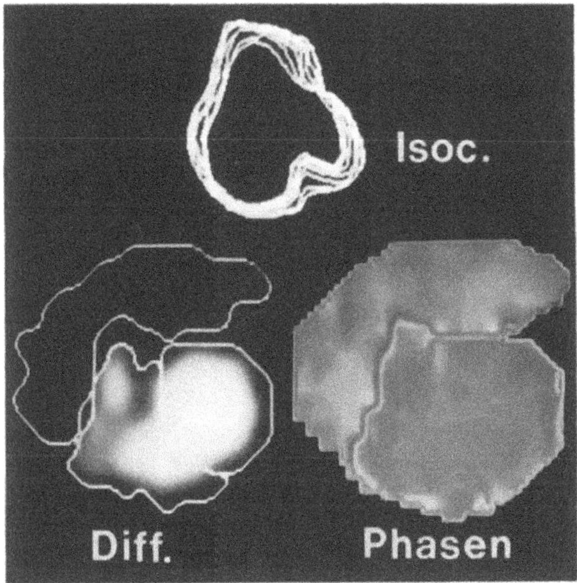

Fig. 7. Analysis of gated blood pool data yields information about various regions of the left ventricle. The difference scan (diff.) displays the extent of regional contraction, with hypokinetic regions appearing as "cold regions" in the scan (see Fig. 11). The phase scan (phasen) visualizes the homogeneity of the contraction process. The normal heart shows synchronous contraction over the area of both ventricles (compare with the phase scans in Figs. 9, 10, 11, and 13). (Isoc. = contours of the contracting heart.)

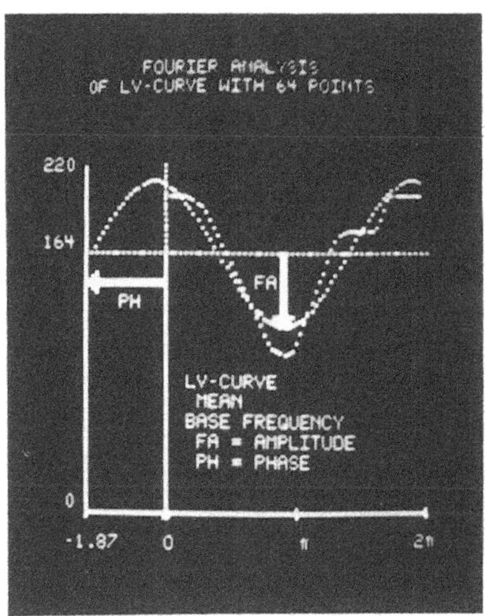

Fig. 8. Fourier analysis. The first Fourier element best fits into the regional time-activity curve. The *amplitude* (FA) corresponds to the extent of contraction (the difference from end-diastole to end-systole). The *phase* (PH) yields information about the coordination of the contraction. Dyskinetic regions show a phase shift as compared with normokinetic regions.

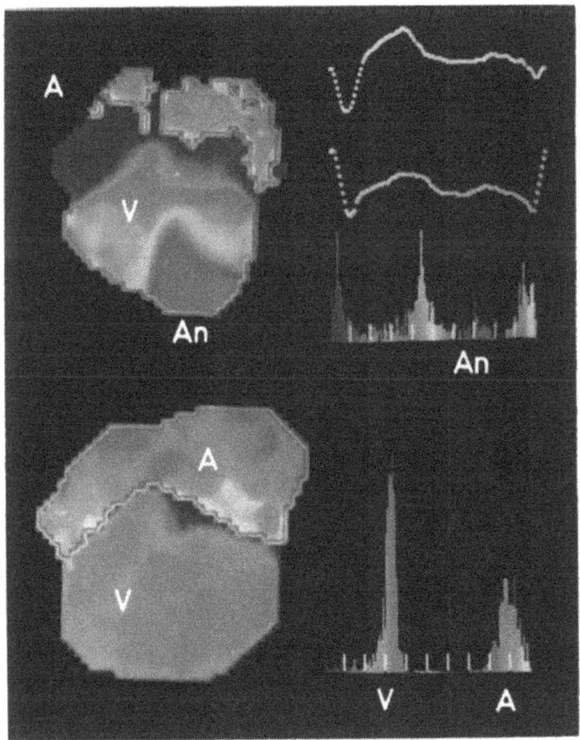

Fig. 9. The phase scan of the normal heart *(lower left)* shows homogeneous contraction of the ventricles (green column *lower right*) and of the atria (pink column *lower right*). A dyskinetic region can be assessed with regard to its size (red region *upper left*) and to the extent of its delay. The phase distribution *(upper right)* shows the dyskinetic (red) region with a delay of 150 msec. (One heart cycle = 600 msec). A = atria and large vessels; An = dyskinetic region; V = ventricles.

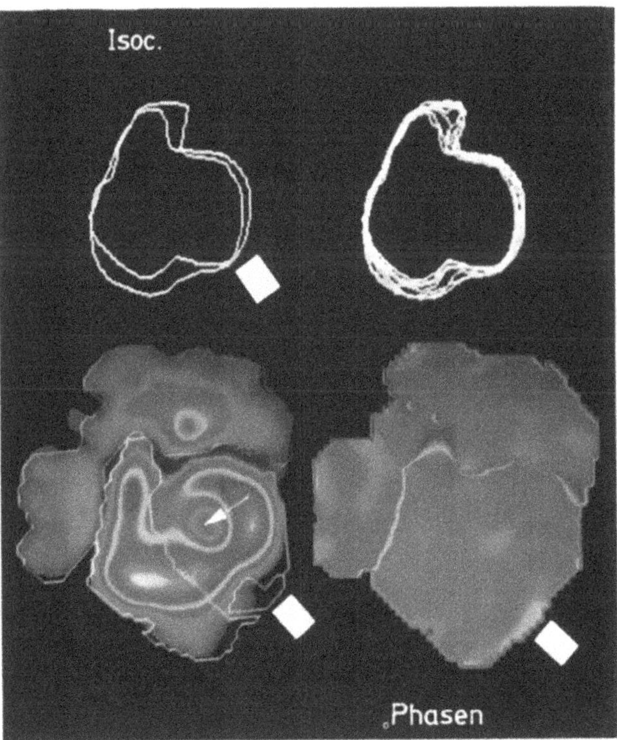

Fig. 10. The importance of a detailed analysis of regional wall motion is demonstrated in a case of anterior wall infarction. The left anterior oblique contour scan shows hypokinesis of the latero-posterior wall and akinesis (square) of the apical region *(upper pictures)*. This diagnosis is corrected by the parametric scans, which demonstrate a hypokinetic region on the left ventricular anteroseptal region (arrow in the amplitude scan *lower left*) and a dyskinetic apical region (phase shift indicated by yellow color in the phase scan *lower right*).

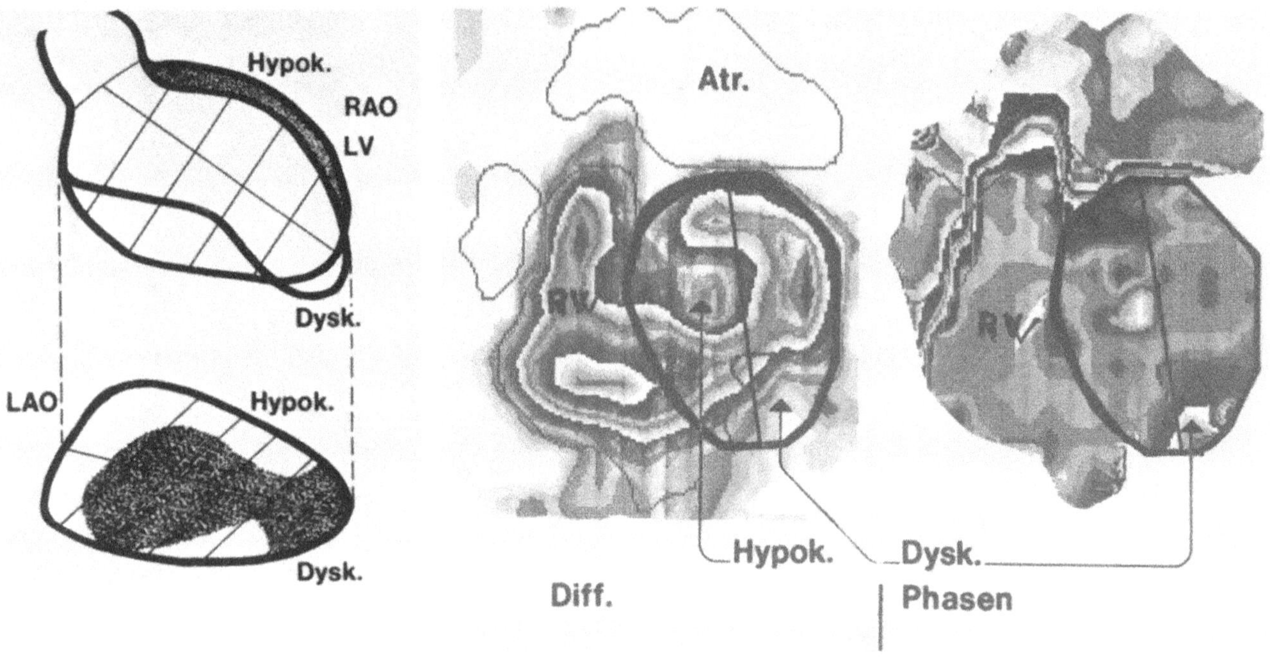

Fig. 11. Patient with anterior wall infarction (identical with Fig. 10). Gray scale plot of parametric scans. The difference scan is similar to the amplitude scan (Fig. 10). The findings correspond to the right anterior oblique ventriculogram *(left picture)*.

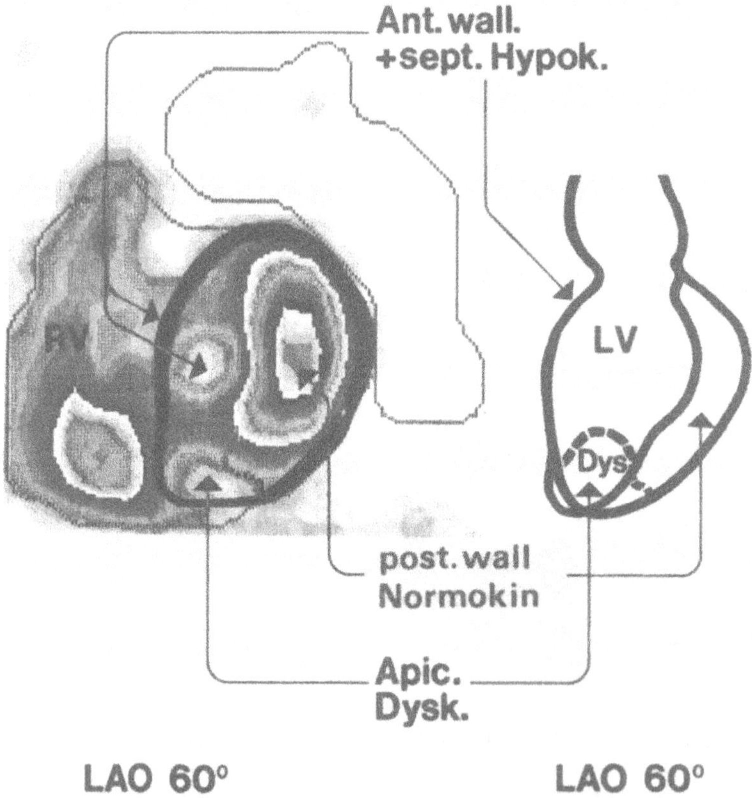

Fig. 12. In the left anterior oblique projection, the anterior and posterior walls overlap. Differentiation is possible in a 60° left anterior oblique projection.

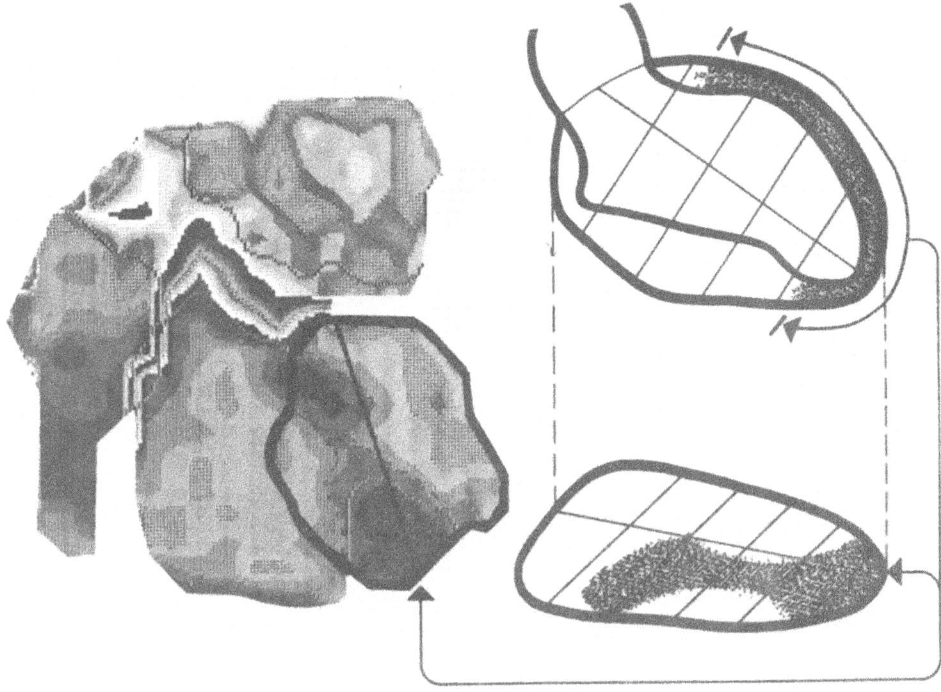

Fig. 13. Anterior wall and apical hypokinesis is present on the contrast ventriculogram, while dyskinesis is also present on the phase scan (*left*).

ysis, the ventricular size is determined by incorporating all elements with an amplitude higher than twice the noise. In our experience, the contour assessment that is usually applied underestimates the size of the left ventricle. The background area chosen as reference is not critical, provided that it is outside the end-systolic left ventricular contour [16, 17]. The subtraction method chosen is important: ejection fraction is underestimated by the usual horizontal plane subtraction method. An inclined plane procedure, which takes into account background inhomogeneity, yields better results (Fig. 6).

Assessment of Regional Wall Motion Abnormalities

Wall-motion abnormalities can be assessed by conventional methods in which lines are drawn to the ventricular contours (median line, hemiaxes) and their diastolic-systolic shortening is measured [36]. As has been explained above, however, this contour-related quantitation procedure, in our opinion, does not take full advantage of the available data. Full exploitation can be achieved by the parametric scan method, which is based on the set of regional time-activity (time-volume) curves of one representative heart cycle (Figs. 1 and 2). Four to six of the parametric scans are usually performed: (1) end-diastolic end-systolic count difference, (2) count difference between end-systole and the end of fast-filling phase, (3) contraction velocity, (4) relaxation velocity, and, after Fourier analysis, the (5) amplitude and (6) phase of the first Fourier element (Figs. 7–13).

Validation of the Technique

Validation of Global Parameters (The Ejection Fraction)

Ejection fraction is the most important global parameter that can be obtained by ECG-gated radionuclide ventriculography. Many studies have found excellent correlation between ejection fraction estimates obtained by ECG-gated ventriculography and by monoplane and biplane ventriculography (r= 0.8–0.97) [10, 12, 20, 28, 36, 39, 48, 50, 51, 55]. The radionuclide procedure systematically underestimates the ejection fraction (regression coefficient about 0.8), partly because the usual subtraction method does not take into account background inhomogeneities. The inclined plane method, in contrast, yields good correlation and good regression [16, 17] (Fig. 6).

Table 1. Regional wall motion assessment: radionuclide vs. contrast ventriculography

Parametric images of the left ventricle	No. of patients	Conformity (%) (four-fold table test)	Correlation coefficient (four-fold table test)	Sensitivity (%)	Specifity (%)	Likelihood ratio
1. Count difference, end-diastole to end-systole	65	84.6	0.67	80.0	95.0	16.0
2. Count difference, end fast-filling period to end-systole	65	90.8	0.76	90.9	90.5	9.6
3. Contraction velocity	67	89.6	0.72	93.5	81.0[a]	10.5
4. Relaxation velocity	67	89.6	0.72	97.8	71.4[a]	3.4
5. Fourier amplitude	67	86.6	0.72	80.4	100.0	∞
6. Fourier phase	66	72.7	0.54	60.0[b]	100.0[b]	∞
7. Combination of parametric scans No. 5 and 6 for detection of regional wall motion abnormalities	65	90.8	0.79	86.4	100.0	∞
8. Combination of parametric scans No. 1, 2, 5 and 6 for detection of regional wall motion abnormalities	68	91.2	0.77	91.5	90.5	9.6
9. Fourier phase scan for detection of dyskinetic regions	65	63.1	0.19	75.0	61.4[c]	1.9

[a] Reference was the extent of contraction estimated by the end-diastolic–end-systolic contrast ventriculograms. For this reason impaired contraction and relaxation velocities with normal extent of contraction are characterised as false positive

[b] Hypokinesis and akinesis detected by contrast ventriculography

[c] Dyskinesis detected by contrast ventriculography

Table 2. Comparison of the relaxation velocity parametric image with contrast ventriculography

Contrast ventriculography	Radionuclide ventriculography (relaxation velocity scan)[a]		
	Normal	Pathologic	Total
Normal	15	6	21
Pathologic	1	45	46
Total	16	51	67

[a] $n=67$

Table 4. Comparison of the Fourier phase parametric image with contrast ventriculography

Contrast ventriculography	Radionuclide ventriculography (Fourier phase scan)[a]		
	Normal	Phase shift	Total
Normal	35	22	57
Dyskinesis	2	6	8
Total	37	28	65

[a] $n=65$

Table 3. Comparison of a combination of parametric images (count differences, end-diastole to end-systole and end-fast-filling period to end-systole; Fourier amplitude; and Fourier phase) with contrast ventriculography

Contrast ventriculography	Radionuclide ventriculography (combination of parametric images)[a]		
	Normal	Pathologic	Total
Normal	19	2	21
Pathologic	4	43	47
Total	23	45	68

$n=68$

Validation of Regional Parameters

The regional curves seem to be of doubtful reliability with respect to motility because of the statistical problems entailed by the small size (0.7 cm^2) of each heart pixel. To control this problem, a parametric scan is constructed that displays the regional correlation – the similarity of the regional time-activity curves in the ventricular area – by comparing the respective curve points. The correlation in the center of the left ventricle is better than 0.9 and in peripheral regions better than 0.75 in the normal heart. Correlation decreases in the area of the right ventricle where the atrium overlaps and in regions with motion abnormalities [2, 5, 16]. Results from about 500 scans have demonstrated the reliability of the regional time-activity curves (see above); thus, the most important prerequisite has been fulfilled for further data processing to obtain parametric scans [2, 5].

Parametric scans (four to six per patient) were compared with biplane contrast ventriculograms in 67 patients with either suspected coronary artery disease or valvular diseases. The left ventricular region of the left anterior oblique radionuclide ventriculogram was divided into seven areas, the right anterior

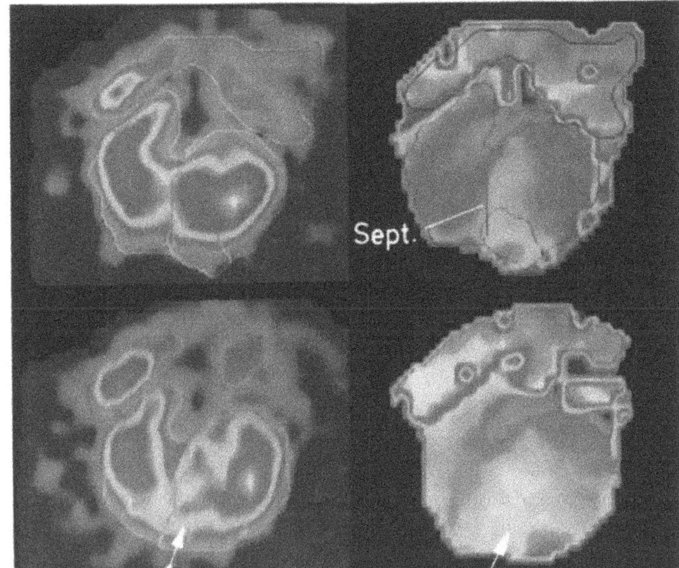

Fig. 14. Patient with stenosis of the left anterior descending artery. Normal extent of contraction at rest *(upper left)*. Under stress (50 W load) the extent of contraction in the anterior and apical region is decreased (arrow, *lower left*). The phase scan reveals the apical and anterior wall region as dyskinetic at rest. Significant extension of the dyskinetic region under stress (arrow, *lower right*). (*Sept.* = septum.)

oblique contrast ventriculogram into nine areas. Of the 536 areas shown in the ventriculogram, 158 (29.3%) showed a wall motion abnormality, which is comparable to the 31.3% abnormal scans found in the radionuclide ventriculogram. Parametric scans vary in the reliability with which they detect regional wall motion abnormalities (Table 1). The relaxation velocity scan is the most sensitive (97.8%). This corresponds to observations that decreased relaxation velocity is the first sign of myocardial insufficiency. The low specificity (six false-positive findings [Table 2]) may result from the fact that the reference method (the end-diastolic – end-systolic contrast ventriculogram) does not permit the determination of velocities. The combination of four parametric scans (Table 3) yields the best results (four false-negative and two false-positive) in 68 investigations. The phase scintigram would appear to be a more sensitive procedure than the contrast ventriculogram: 22 patients without dyskinesis in the contrast ventriculogram revealed significant regional phase shifting (Table 4).

Clinical Applications and Results

Radionuclide ventriculography as a noninvasive method to assess cardiac dynamics and ventricular wall motion at rest and during exercise has its principal application in screening and follow-up of patients with suspected coronary artery disease, with or without infarction [5, 6, 10–12, 15, 18, 19, 23, 25, 30, 36, 37, 39, 40, 43, 46, 47, 52, 53, 55, and M. Stauch et al., unpublished data]. Though the majority of patients with suspected acute myocardial infarction do not represent a diagnostic problem, the parametric scans can give additional information concerning site, extent, and mode of regional wall motion abnormalities and their impact on left ventricular function. Follow-up investigations often show a return to normal motion or transition to an aneurysm. Radionuclide ventriculography is complementary to perfusion scintigraphy because contractility is extremely sensitive to reductions in coronary blood flow. Detection of subacute and chronic infarctions by radionuclide ventriculography was possible in more than 90% of cases, while thallium scintigraphy detected only 66% of old infarctions [48].

The high sensitivity of contractility to coronary blood flow reduction during stress enables accurate detection of patients with coronary artery stenosis [10]. Patients with substantial coronary artery obstruction show a maximal dilatation of the microcirculation distal to the lesion. The coronary reserve is exhausted, and further dilatation is not possible when the patient exercises. As a result, increased oxygen demand is not met, and the regional ischemia causes altered ventricular contraction, with decreased ejection fraction and regional dyskinesis (Fig. 14).

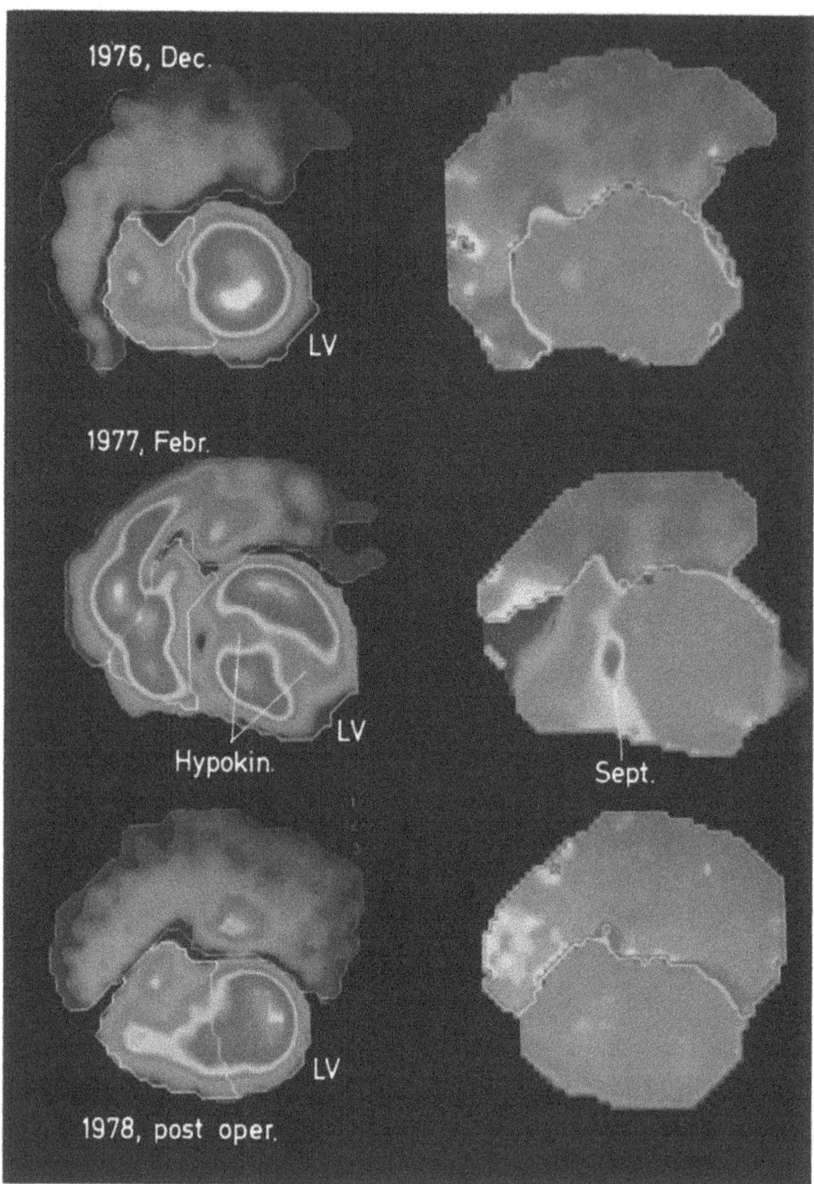

Fig. 15. Patient with aortic valve insufficiency. A moderately increased size of the left ventricle is evident on the Dec. 1976 images. The amplitude scan *(upper left)* shows good contraction in the left ventricular area. The phase scan *(upper right)* demonstrates good co-ordination of the contraction in both ventricles. Two months later (Febr. 1977) there was dilatation of the left ventricle with regional hypokinesis (Hypokin.) and dyskinesis in the septal region (Sept.). After surgery (1978, post oper.) the left ventricle was normal in size and contractility.

With stress scintigraphy the sensitivity and specificity for the detection of coronary artery disease was better than 90% in such patients [10, 19]. In these studies, the global ejection fraction was measured and assessments of regional motility were made qualitatively from the radionuclide cineventriculogram. Other studies have shown a decreased rate of change in global volume in patients with coronary artery disease [22, 49]. Myocardial relaxation is a particularly sensitive indicator of impending myocardial insufficiency. Breuel et al. analyzed the left ventricular time-volume curve in 23 normal subjects and in 27 patients with coronary artery disease under rest conditions [12]. No difference was found between the two groups in ejection fraction and contraction velocity, but significantly decreased relaxation velocity occurred in the coronary artery disease group. This is in agreement with our own results (Geffers et al., unpublished data) and with Hirakawa et al. [23].

But are those early alterations in the global left

ventricular time-volume curve also demonstrable in the regional curves? In the case of decreased relaxation velocity, the corresponding relaxation velocity scan should reveal an abnormal region before the amplitude scan becomes positive. In fact, the relaxation velocity scan seems to show the highest sensitivity in detecting regional wall motion abnormalities (Table 1). Unfortunately, the difference between these and other parametric scans did not prove statistically significant. Thus, a reliable assessment of the additional diagnostic value of quantitative evaluation procedures is not possible at the present time.

Radionuclide ventriculography is useful in many areas. It can be used to visualize the entire profile of the interventricular septum, which shows characteristic alterations in cases of hypertropic cardiomyopathy [41, 45, 47]. Because the investigation can be repeated within several hours without an additional radiation dose, it lends itself to heart function investigations under varying pharmaceutical and physiological interventions [10, 11, 19, 25, 47, 49]. Follow-up studies [14, 15, 19, 41] can demonstrate the progress of heart failure (Fig. 15). While the first-transit method is clearly superior to the gated blood pool procedure for the investigation of valvular disease, aortic and mitral valve insufficiency can be measured by the ratio of the left and right ventricular end-diastolic–end-systolic count differences, with good agreement with the angiographic estimates ($r = 0.79$) (H. Geffers et al., unpublished data).

Comparison between Equilibrium and First-Transit Ventriculography

Radionuclide ventriculography after homogeneous tracer distribution is superior to the first-transit technique in several ways:

1. The injection technique is not critical.

2. Because of the lower count rate, the investigation can be performed without count loss even with cameras of low sensitivity.

3. Lower count rates can be compensated for by increasing the imaging time, thus improving the counting statistics.

4. Follow-up investigations under stress, after drug administration, and in various positions are possible without additional injection and additional radiation exposure.

The method is inferior to the first-transit procedure in the following ways:

1. Right and left ventricular differentiation is only possible in the left anterior oblique projection. Detailed analysis of the right ventricle is not possible (Fig. 4).

2. The investigation is time consuming (4–15 minutes).

3. Transit times and corresponding information important to the evaluation of valvular failure cannot be obtained.

A combination of both procedures gives the most information.

Conclusions

1. Radionuclide ventriculography after homogenous tracer distribution provides a reliable noninvasive method for the global and regional assessment of left ventricular function.

2. The most important global parameter is the left ventricular ejection fraction, which can be measured accurately. Decrease of ejection fraction during exercise is an important feature of coronary artery disease. Maximal relaxation velocity (fast filling phase) measured from the global time-volume curve, seems to be the most sensitive global parameter of left ventricular insufficiency.

3. Regional wall motion abnormalities can be assessed qualitatively from the cineventriculogram ("movie mode") or in a quantitative manner. During stress, hypokinetic, dyskinetic, and akinetic regions are characteristic features of coronary artery disease.

4. The most extensive quantitative evaluation of regional wall motion is based on the regional time-activity curve of the representative heart cycle, which can be obtained reliably. Checking the set of regional time-activity curves with respect to one parameter results in a parametric scan, which displays the distribution of the respective parameter in the left ventricular region.

5. In our department, six parametric scans including distribution of amplitude and phase of the first Fourier element are obtained. These six scans describe the regional wall motion reliably and in detail. While determination of ejection fraction and qualitative assessment of regional wall motion has been widely applied, the clinical value of the parametric scans cannot be finally assessed at this time.

Acknowledgment. The authors are indebted to Informatique Ltd. for the generous support of this work.

References

1. Adam, W.E., Bitter, F., Lorenz, W.J.: Der Computer als Hilfsmittel zur Verbesserung der nuklearmedizinischen Funktionsdiagnostik. In: Computers in Radiology, edited by R. de Haene and A. Wambersie. Basel, Karger, 1970, pp. 459–464
2. Adam, W.E., Geffers, H., Sigel, H., Bitter, F., Kampmann, H., Stauch, M., Wassermann, B.: Evaluation of left ventricular function by radionuclide angiography. Herz 2:195–199, 1977
3. Adam, W.E., Meyer, G., Bitter, F., Kampmann, H., Stauch, M., Paiva, M.: Camera-kinematography: A nuclear medicine procedure for imaging heart kinetics. J. Nucl. Biol. Med. 18:53–59, 1974
4. Adam, W.E., Schenck, P., Kampmann, H., Lorenz, W.J., Schneider, W.G., Ammann, W., Bilaniuk, L.: Investigation of cardiac dynamics using scintillation camera and computer. In: Medical Radioisotope Scintigraphy II, Vienna, IAEA, 1969, pp. 77–89
5. Adam, W.E., Sigel, H., Geffers, H., Kampmann, H., Bitter, F., Stauch, M.: Analyse der regionalen Wandbewegung des linken Ventrikels bei koronarer Herzerkrankung durch ein nichtinvasives Verfahren (Radionuclid-Kinematographie). Z. Kardiol. 66:545–555, 1977
6. Ashburn, W.L., Kostuk, W.J., Karliner, J.S., Peterson, K.L., Sobel, B.E.: Left ventricular volume and ejection fraction determination by radionuclide angiography. Semin. Nucl. Med. 3:165–176, 1973
7. Bacharach, S.L., Green, M.V., Borer, J.S., Ostrow, H.G., Redwood, D.R., Johnston, G.S.: ECG-gated scintillation probe measurement of left ventricular function. J. Nucl. Med. 18:1176–1183, 1977
8. Bitter, F., Adam, W.E., Kampmann, H., Meyer, G., Weller, R.: Automated selection of areas of interest in dynamic studies and camera-kinematography of the heart. Proceedings of the Fifth Symposium on Sharing of Computer Programs and Technology in Nuclear Medicine. Salt Lake City, 1975, pp. 48–60
9. Bitter, F., Besch, W., Schäfer, N., Sigmund, E.: Integrierte Herz-Kreislauf-Analyse mit Hilfe der quantitativen Funktionsszintigraphie. In: Frontiers of Nuclear Medicine, edited by W. Horst. Berlin, New York, Springer, 1971, pp. 250–261
10. Borer, J.S., Bacharach, S.L., Green, M.V., Kent, K.M., Epstein, S.E., Johnston, G.S.: Real-time radionuclide cineangiography in the non-invasive evaluation of global and regional left ventricular function at rest and during exercise in patients with coronary-artery disease. N. Engl. J. Med. 296:839–844, 1977
11. Borer, J.S., Bacharach, S.L., Green, M.V., Kent, K.M., Johnston, G.S., Epstein, S.E.: Effect of nitroglycerin on exercise-induced abnormalities of left ventricular regional function and ejection fraction in coronary artery disease: Assessment by radionuclide cineangiography in symptomatic and asymptomatic patients. Circulation 57:314–320, 1978
12. Breuel, H.-P., Felix, R., Knopp, R., Otten, H., Simon, H., Winkler, C.: Funktionsszintigraphie der Kontraktion des linken Ventrikels. ROEFO 129:317–320, 1978
13. Breuel, H.-P., Knopp, R., Felix, R., Neumann, G.P., Altland, H., Winkler, C.: Funktionsszintigraphie der Kontraktion des linken Ventrikels. II. Methodische Untersuchungen zur Background-Korrektur. ROEFO 129:18–23, 1978
14. Brill, G., Oberhausen, E., Klein, C.P.: Nuklearmedizinische Bestimmung der Ejektionsfraktion, des Herzminutenvolumens und zeitlichen Volumen-Differentials. Nuklearmedizin 17:199–202, 1978
15. Bulkley, B.H., Hutchins, G.M., Bailey, I., Strauss, H.W., Pitt, B.: Thallium 201 imaging and gated cardiac blood pool scans in patients with ischemic and idiopathic congestive cardiomyopathy: A clinical and pathologic study. Circulation 55:753–760, 1977
16. Geffers, H., Adam, W.E., Bitter, F., Sigel, H., Kampmann, H.: Data processing and functional imaging in radionuclide ventriculography. 4. International Cinference on Data Processing and Medical Imaging. Nashville, Tenn., June 1977
17. Geffers, H., Adam, W.E., Bitter, F., Sigel, H., Stauch, M.: Radionuklid-Ventrikulographie. I. Grundlagen und Methoden. Nuklearmedizin 17:206–210, 1978
18. Geffers, H., Sigel, H., Bitter, F., Kampmann, H., Stauch, M., Adam, W.E.: Untersuchungen der segmentalen Wandbewegung des linken Ventrikels bei Herzgesunden und Myokardinfarktpatienten mit einer katheterlosen nulkearmedizinischen Methode (Kamera-Kinematographie des Herzens). Z. Kardiol. 65:680–692, 1976
19. Green, M.V., Borer, J.S., Bacharach, S.L.: Radionuclide cineangiography during stress. Nuklearmedizin 17:229–231, 1978
20. Green, M.V., Brody, W.R., Douglas, M.A., Borer, J.S., Ostrow, H.G., Line, B.R., Bacharach, S.L., Johnston, G.S.: Ejection fraction by count rate from gated images. J. Nucl. Med. 19: 880–883, 1978
21. Green, M.V., Ostrow, H.G., Douglas, M.A., Myers, R.W., Scott, R.N., Bailey, J.J., Johnston, G.S.: High-temporal-resolution ECG-gated scintigraphic angiocardiography. J. Nucl. Med. 16:95–98, 1975
22. Hammermeister, K.E., Warbasse, J.R.: The rate of change of left ventricular volume in man. II. Diastolic events in health and disease. Circulation 49:739–747, 1974
23. Hirakawa, A., Saito, M., Motohara, S., Matsumura, T., Sakurai, T., Kadota, K., Yamada, N., Hara, A., Ogino, K., Kawai, C., Kuwahara, M.: Decreased early diastolic dV/dt in ischemic heart disease observed by ECG-gated radiocardiography. Jap. Circ. J. 41:507–514, 1977
24. Hoffmann, C., Kleine, N.: Eine neue Methode zur unblutigen Messung des Schlagvolumens am Menschen über viele Tage mit Hilfe von radioaktiven Isotopen. Verh. Dtsch. Ges. Kreislaufforsch. 31:93–96, 1965
25. Holman, B.L.: Promising new radiotracer technics for the diagnosis of coronary-artery disease. N. Engl. J. Med. 296:876–877, 1977
26. Hundeshagen, H.: Die digitale Radionuklid-Angiokardiographie. In: Nuklearmedizin: Fortschritte der Nuklearmedizin in klinischer und technologischer Sicht, edited by H.W. Pabst, G. Hör, H.A.E. Schmidt. Stuttgart, F.K. Schattauer, 1975, pp 17–26
27. Hundeshagen, H.: Radiokardiographie. Grundlagen und Entwicklung einer Methode. Heidelberg, A. Hüthig, 1970
28. Klein, C., Brill, G., Oberhausen, E., Bette, L.: Radiokardiographische Bestimmung des Herzminutenvolumens und der Ejectionsfraktion. Ein Vergleich mit konventionellen kardiologischen Untersuchungsverfahren. Z. Kardiol. 67:92–98, 1978
29. Knopp, R., Breuel, H.-P., Schmidt, H., Winkler, C.: Funktionsszintigraphie des Herzens. I. Datentechnische Grundlagen und Methodik. ROEFO 128:44–47, 1978
30. Lenaers, A., Lequime, J.: Radioactive isotope in the diagnosis of heart disease. Acta Cardiol. 33:205–218, 1978
31. Loken, M.K., Medina, J.R., Lillehei, J.F., L'Heureux, P.L., Kush, G.S., Ebert, R.V.: Regional pulmonary function evaluation using xenon-133, a scintillation camera and computer. Radiology 93:1261–1266, 1969
32. Luig, H., Emrich, D.: Fortschritte bei der nicht invasiven Registrierung volumenäquivalenter Kurven des linken Ventrikels mit einer nucklearmedizinischen Methodik. Herz 2:200–201, 1977
33. Luig, H., Emrich, D., Breuel, H.-P., Strauer, B.-E., Neubaur, J., Kisselbach, V.J.: Non-invasive determination of volume-equivalent curves of the left ventricle. In: Dynamic Studies

with Radioisotopes in Medicine. Vienna, I.A.E.A., 1975, pp. 207–217

34. Luig, H., Lahne, R., Domovitz, S.: Ein Datensystem für kardiologische Untersuchungen mit einer Gammakamera. Medizinische Physik 2:99–112, 1977
35. MayIntyre, W.J., Christie, J.H.: A comparison of data averaging of radioisotope scan data by photographic and dimensional computer techniques. In: Medical Radioisotope Scintigraphy I, Vienna, I.A.E.A. 1969, pp. 771–781
36. Ogris, E., Pachinger, O., Sochor, H., Probst, P., Joskowicz, G., Kaindl, F.: Assessment of regional wall motion in coronary artery disease using radionuclide methods. Nuklearmedizin 17:221–224, 1978
37. Parisi, A.F., Tow, D.E., Sasahara, A.A.: Clinical appraisal of current nuclear and other noninvasive cardiac diagnostic techniques. Am. J Cardiol. 38:722–730, 1976
38. Parisi, A.F., Tow, D.E., Felix, W.R., Jr., Sasahara, A.A.: Noninvasive cardiac diagnosis. N. Engl. J. Med. 296:427–432, 1977
39. Parker, J.A., Uren, R.F., Jones, A.G., Maddox, D.E., Zimmerman, R.E., Neill, J.M., Holman, B.L.: Radionuclide left ventriculography with the slant hole collimator. J. Nucl. Med. 18:848–851, 1977
40. Pitt, B., Strauss, H.W.: Myocardial imaging in the noninvasive evaluation of patients with suspected ischemic heart disease. Am. J. Cardiol. 37:797–806, 1976
41. Pitt, B., Strauss, H.W.: Myocardial perfusion imaging and gated cardiac blood pool scanning: Clinical application. Am. J. Cardiol. 38:739–746, 1976
42. Pitt, B., Strauss, H.W.: Cardiovascular nuclear medicine. Semin. Nucl. Med. 7:3–6, 1977
43 Planiol, T., Itti, R., Pottier, J.M., Pourcelot, L., Brochier, M., Morand, P.: The contribution of nuclear medicine and ultrasound in cardiac surgery. Acta Cardiol. 33:339–370, 1978
44. Pohost, G.M., Pastore, J.O., McKusick, K.A., Chiotellis, P.N., Kapellakis, G.Z., Myers, G.S., Dinsmore, R.E., Block, P.C.: Detection of left atrial myxoma by gated radionuclide cardiac imaging. Circulation 55:88–92, 1977
45. Pohost, G.M., Vignola, P.A., McKusick, K.E., Block, P.C., Myers, G.S., Walker, H.J., Copen, D.L., Dinsmore, R.E.: Hypertrophic cardiomyopathy: Evaluation by gated cardiac blood pool scanning. Circulation 55:92–99, 1977
46. Qureshi, S., Wagner, H.N., Jr., Alderson, P.O., Housholder, D.F., Douglas, K.H., Lotter, M.G., Nickoloff, E.L., Tanabe, M., Knowles, L.G.: Evaluation of left-ventricular function in normal persons and patients with heart disease. J. Nucl. Med. 19:135–141, 1978
47. Sauer, E., Sebening, H., Lutilsky, L., Dressler, H., Hör, G., Pabst, H.W., Blömer, H.: Die Beurteilung der globalen und regionalen linksventrikulären Funktion in Ruhe und während Ergometerbelastung bei Patienten mit koronarer Herzkrankheit mit der EKG-getriggerten Herzbinnenraumszintigraphie. Nuklearmedizin 17:225–228, 1978
48. Sigel, H., Adam, W.E., Geffers, H., Bitter, F., Stauch, M.: Radionuklid-Ventrikulographie. III. Klinische Ergebnisse: Parameter der regionalen Wandbewegung. Nuklearmedizin 17:216–220, 1978
49. Spiller, P.: Quantitative Lävokardiographie. München, Urban und Schwarzenberg, 1978
50. Stauch, M., Sigel, H., Geffers, H., Bitter, F., Adam, W.E.: Noninvasive determination of the left ventricular ejection fraction with radionuclides. In: Computers in Cardiology, edited by H.G. Ostrow and K.L. Ripley. Long Beach, 1977, p. 181
51. Stauch, M., Sigel, H., Geffers, H., Gerst, C.M., Bitter, F., Adam, W.E.: Radionuklid-Ventrikulographie. II. Klinische Ergebnisse: Parameter der globalen Ventrikelfunktion. Nuclearmedizin 17:211–215, 1978
52. Strauss, H.W., Pitt, B.: Cardiovascular nuclear medicine: Its role in patients with coronary heart disease. Appl. Radiol. 57–61, 1975
53. Strauss, H.W., Pitt, B.: Common procedures for the noninvasive determination of regional myocardial perfusion, evaluation of regional wall motion and detection of acute infarction. Am. J. Cardiol. 38:731–738, 1976
54. Strauss, H.W., Pitt, B.: Evaluation of cardiac function and structure with radioactive tracer techniques. Circulation 57:645–654, 1978
55. Strauss, H.W., Zaret, B.L., Hurley, P.J., Natarajan, T.K., Pitt, B.: A scintiphotographic method for measuring left ventricular ejection fraction in man without cardiac catheterization. Am. J. Cardiol. 28:575–580, 1971
56. Wagner, H.N., Jr., Wake, R., Nickoloff, E., Natarajan, T.K.: The nuclear stethoscope: A simple device for generation of left ventricular volume curves. Am. J. Cardiol. 38:747–750, 1976
57. Zaret, B.L., Strauss, H.W., Hurley, P.J., Natarajan, T.K., Pitt, B.: A noninvasive scintiphotographic method for detecting regional ventricular dysfunction in man. N. Engl. J. Med. 28:1165–1170. 1971

Myocardial Scintigraphy with Infarct-Avid Tracers

B.L. Holman and J. Wynne
Departments of Radiology and Medicine, Harvard Medical School, Boston, Massachusetts, USA

The scintigraphic appearance of infarcted myocardium as an area of increased activity has considerable appeal, since standard techniques, including serum enzyme tests, electrocardiography, and vectorcardiography, provide only indirect evidence of the presence, size, and location of infarcted myocardium. Although these techniques are usually accurate in detecting infarction, the availability of techniques to localize precisely the site of damaged myocardium and the extent of damage is limited. Radiopharmaceuticals that are extracted by normal myocardium, such as potassium and its analogues [1] and radiolabeled fatty acids [2], offer additional help by outlining poorly perfused tissue as regions of decreased tracer concentration in myocardial scans [3]. These radiopharmaceuticals, however, do not permit differentiation of acute infarction and fibrotic or previously infarcted tissue. To overcome these difficulties, investigators have sought agents that accumulate selectively in damaged myocardium.

Technetium-99m Tetracycline

Technetium-99m tetracycline was the first radiopharmaceutical that was found to show infarct avidity in man [4, 5]. Initial results demonstrated that acute myocardial infarction could be detected accurately 24 hours after the injection of ^{99m}Tc-tetracycline [5].

The major limitation to acute infarct scintigraphy with ^{99m}Tc-tetracycline is its slow clearance from the blood, which necessitates a 24-hour delay before imaging can be performed. In addition, because tracer concentration within the infarct is only moderately elevated, uptake in the diaphragmatic segment of the heart may be obscured by the high concentration within the liver.

Technetium-99m Pyrophosphate

At the present time, ^{99m}Tc-pyrophosphate is the radiotracer of choice for imaging acute myocardial infarction in man [6–8]. Fifty percent of the injected dose is extracted by bone and the remainder is rapidly excreted through the kidneys. At 90 minutes, less than 5% of the injected dose remains in the blood.

^{99m}Tc-pyrophosphate uptake is dependent on three factors: local blood flow, calcification, and tissue damage. The uptake of ^{99m}Tc-pyrophosphate is directly related to the degree of tissue damage, but because the pharmaceutical must get to the damaged tissue to be extracted, uptake is inversely related to the extent of flow reduction at low flow. Following acute coronary occlusion, increased concentrations of ^{99m}Tc-pyrophosphate are found in regions with only minimal reductions in blood flow [9]. The highest concentration ratios between damaged and normal myocardium occur when local blood flow is 20–40% of normal. As flow is reduced further, the concentration ratios begin to fall until, in regions of minimal flow (0–5% of normal), ^{99m}Tc-pyrophosphate concentration may be normal.

Observing that hydroxyapatite crystals were formed within mitochondria in the peripheral zones of the acute infarct, Bonte et al. hypothesized that ^{99m}Tc-pyrophosphate, a calcium chelate, is sequestered by these crystals during the acute phase of myocardial infarction [8]. Mitochondrial calcification has been detected as early as two to four hours after permanent occlusion and becomes marked by

Supported in part by USPHS grant HL 17739. Dr. Holman is an Established Investigator of the American Heart Association

Address reprint requests to: B. Leonard Holman, M.D., Department of Radiology, Harvard Medical School, 25 Shattuck Street, Boston, MA 02115, USA

12 to 24 hours [10]. The calcification occurred primarily in irreversibly damaged tissue.

Recent experimental evidence suggests that, while the mechanism for localization may be related to the presence of calcium, the site of sequestration of the radiopharmaceutical is not the mitochondria [11, 12]. Furthermore, doubt has been cast on the precise role of calcification in ^{99m}Tc-pyrophosphate sequestration. Using a fetal mouse heart tissue culture model, Schelbert et al. found a poor correlation between calcium and ^{99m}Tc-pyrophosphate uptake [13].

Technique and Interpretation

Patients suspected of having sustained an acute myocardial infarction are usually admitted directly to the coronary care unit. Because they are usually at risk for developing either electrophysiologic or hemodynamic complications, imaging must be performed at the bedside using portable scintillation cameras.

Routine imaging is performed three hours after the intravenous injection of 10–15 mCi of ^{99m}Tc-pyrophosphate. Images are obtained in the anterior, left anterior oblique, and left lateral projections, with at least 400,000 counts collected in each projection. Multiple projections permit accurate localization of the infarct and separate infarct uptake from overlying bone in equivocal cases.

Parkey et al. developed a grading system for interpretation of ^{99m}Tc-pyrophosphate images that depends on the intensity of the activity over the myocardium [7]. Scintigrams are graded from 0 to 4+. A grade of 0 means that there is no activity in the region of the heart and indicates a negative myocardial scintigram; 1+ is possible but not absolutely definite activity and is also considered to represent a negative scintigram; 2+ is definite but faint activity and indicates an abnormal myocardial scintigram; 3+ and 4+ represent definite and increased activity within the myocardial image. In those scintiscans that are considered positive (2+, 3+, and 4+), the area of increased uptake is also described (anterior, inferior, lateral, or true posterior). While this classification has proved useful, it suffers from shortcomings. Grading is highly subjective and prone to interobserver error. It also does not take into account the difference in accuracy when uptake is focal or diffuse.

In an effort to provide a more objective basis for the interpretation of ^{99m}Tc-pyrophosphate scintigraphy, and in an effort to address the differences both in diagnostic accuracy and in prognosis between diffuse and focal patterns, we have developed an alternative classification [14]. The scintigraphic patterns are divided into the following types (Fig. 1):

A: Normal; myocardial uptake equal to that over the right hemithorax (no identification of a discrete cardiac silhouette);

B_1: Mild diffuse; myocardial uptake exceeding uptake over right hemithorax but less intense than the ribs and distributed over most or all of the myocardium;

B_2: Moderate diffuse; myocardial uptake equal to or greater than the intensity of the ribs but less intense than the sternum;

C: Focal; discrete myocardial uptake less intense than the sternum;

D: Focal; discrete myocardial uptake involving less than 50% of the cardiac silhouette (as estimated from the admission chest radiograph) and equal to or more intense than the sternum;

E: Massive; increase in myocardial uptake involving 50% or more of the cardiac silhouette and equal to or more intense than the sternum.

When myocardial uptake is focal, it can be localized to one or more wall segments from an analysis of the scintigrams obtained in multiple projections. The inferior and lateral wall segments are perpendicular to the detector in the anterior projection while the inferior, true posterior, and anterior segments are perpendicular in the lateral projection (Fig. 2). Frequently, multiple wall segments are involved, since coronary anatomy is variable and the coronary arteries overlap the artificial boundaries defined by these ventricular wall segments.

The accuracy of acute infarct detection with ^{99m}Tc-pyrophosphate imaging has been investigated by a large number of groups over the past five years [6, 14–19]. The greatest sensitivity for the detection of acute myocardial infarction is between 16 hours and six days after the onset of symptoms. The sensitivity of the technique, that is, the percentage of patients with acute infarction who have abnormal scintigrams, ranges from 59% to 100%. The composite sensitivity for all patients in these studies is 92%. The incidence of abnormal scintigrams in patients without evidence of acute infarction is 18%.

The time at which imaging is performed after injection affects the specificity of the test. When imaging is performed 90 minutes after injection, only 55% of patients who show diffuse myocardial uptake prove to have an acute infarction [14]. Other patterns, however, are more accurate. In our series, none of the 21 patients with a normal pattern 90 minutes after injection had an acute infarction. Eighty percent of patients with focal uptake had acute infarctions as did all patients with massive uptake. By delaying scintig-

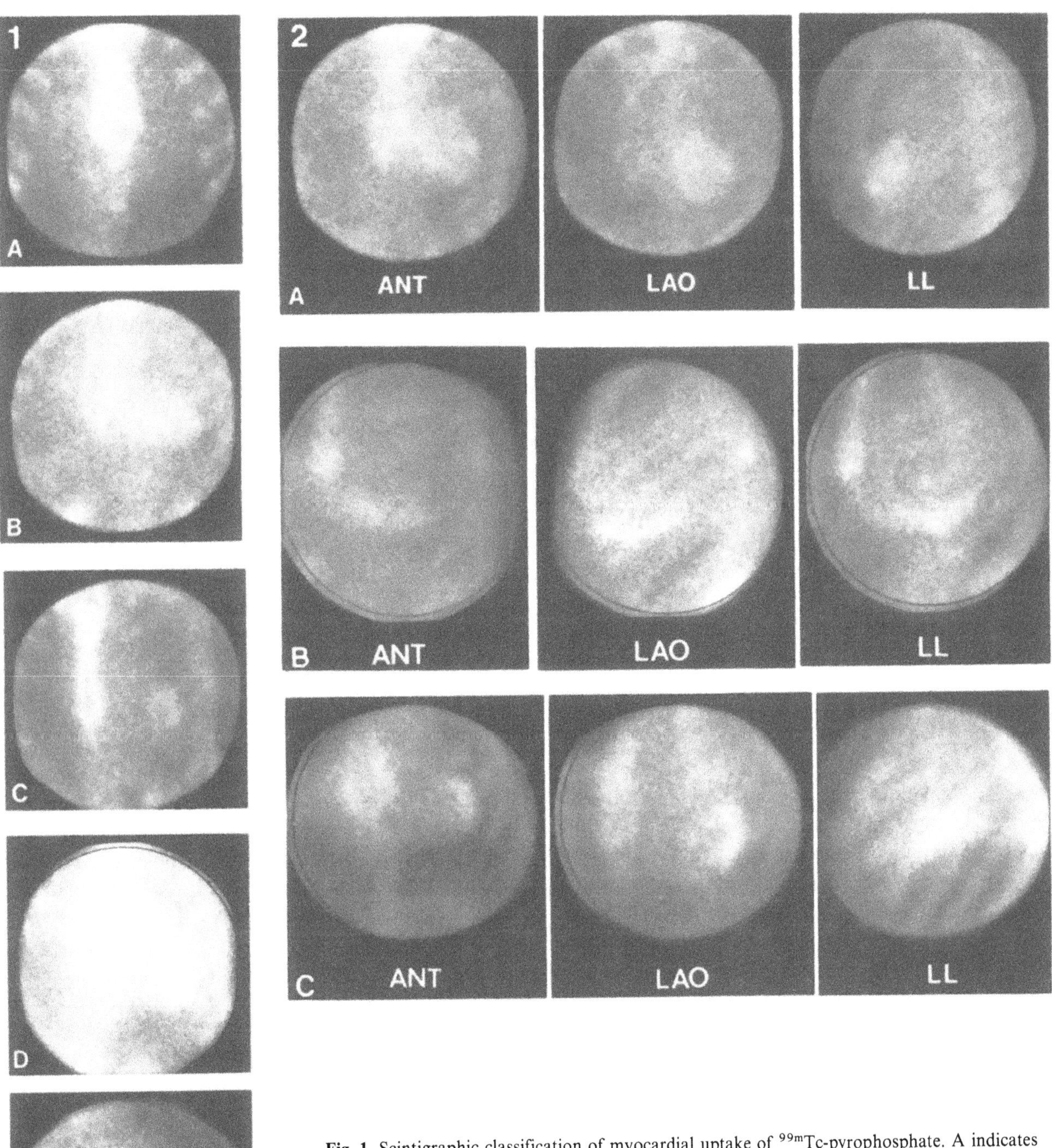

Fig. 1. Scintigraphic classification of myocardial uptake of ^{99m}Tc-pyrophosphate. A indicates normal uptake; B diffuse; C focal, less intense than the sternum; and E massive. (Reprinted with permission from [6].)

Fig. 2A–C. A Myocardial scintigraphy with ^{99m}Tc-pyrophosphate in patients with acute anterior myocardial infarct (ANT indicates an anterior projection, LAO left anterior oblique, and LL left lateral). **B** Myocardial scintigraphy in a patient with an acute inferior myocardial infarct. Note posterior wall extension. **C** Myocardial scintigraphy in a patient with an acute lateral myocardial infarct.

raphy until three hours after injection, the specificity of the diffuse pattern can be increased. Seventy-five percent of patients with diffuse uptake equal to or greater in intensity than the ribs at three hours had acute infarction. On the other hand, faint diffuse uptake is indeterminate for the diagnosis of acute myocardial infarction regardless of the time interval between injection and imaging, since over 20% of patients with this pattern at either 90 minutes or three hours had acute infarction.

While the technique is most sensitive between 16 hours and six days after the onset of symptoms, acute infarction can be detected as early as four hours after the onset of symptoms [20]. The detection rate is somewhat lower with early imaging. Eleven of 15 patients with acute infarction showed abnormal scintigraphic results between four and eight hours after symptoms began. In all cases the uptake was faint to moderate in intensity and focal in distribution. In five of the 11 cases, the serum creatine phosphokinase activity was within normal limits at the time scintigraphy was performed. Three of the four patients with normal images had massive transmural infarctions with symptoms of severe pump failure. Repeat scintigraphy was abnormal in the two patients surviving to 24 hours after infarction.

Patients with uncomplicated acute myocardial infarction show peak ^{99m}Tc-pyrophosphate uptake between 48 and 72 hours after onset of symptoms. After this time, the intensity of uptake decreases, reaching normal levels after one to two weeks. In many patients, however, the scintigraphic pattern returns to normal very slowly. Olson et al. observed a return to normal in only 43% of patients six to 37 weeks after acute infarction [21]. Forty-seven percent of the patients demonstrated improved but still abnormal scintigraphic results, while only 6% of the scintigrams remained unchanged. In 4%, the intensity worsened. In patients with persistently abnormal scintigrams, the pattern was usually mildly diffuse. Only 20% of these patients had focal activity. While some had developed ventricular aneurysms, the majority of such patients studied postmortem only had evidence of fibrosis, myocytolysis, and significant myocardial degeneration.

The failure of ^{99m}Tc-pyrophosphate scintigraphy to return to normal within one to two weeks in the majority of patients with acute infarction limits the specificity of the technique in patients with recent myocardial infarction and recurrent symptoms. In patients with infarction who return with recurring symptoms, a single study at the time that reinfarction is suspected is of value only if it is negative or intensely positive. Sequential scintigraphy is of value if the scintigraphic pattern follows a classic course after the recurrent symptoms. If the intensity of pyrophosphate uptake increases for the first 48 to 72 hours with subsequent rapid decrease in intensity, the probability of reinfarction is high. In all other cases, acute myocardial infarction cannot be distinguished from recent infarction without a baseline study at the time of the initial infarction.

A number of conditions other than acute infarction can also cause increased myocardial uptake of ^{99m}Tc-pyrophosphate (Table 1). Several investigators have observed abnormal scintigrams in patients with unstable angina pectoris but without clinical evidence of acute infarction [15, 23, 24, 38, 39]. The pattern is usually mildly diffuse.

Table 1. Differential diagnosis of ^{99m}Tc-pyrophosphate myocardial uptake

1. Acute myocardial infarction
2. Recent large myocardial infarction [21, 22]
3. Ventricular aneurysm [23]
4. Unstable angina pectoris [24, 25]
5. Cardiomyopathy [23]
6. Cardioversion [26]
7. Myocardial contusion [27]
8. Breast tumor [28]
9. Metastatic carcinoma
10. Adriamycin toxicity [29]
11. Valvular calcification [30, 31]
12. Skin lesions [32]
13. Rib fracture [33, 34]
14. Calcified costal cartilage [35]
15. Abdominal activity
16. Blood pool activity [36, 37]

Diffuse and focal patterns of increased ^{99m}Tc-pyrophosphate uptake have been observed in patients with idiopathic cardiomyopathy [40], ventricular aneurysms [23], and valvular calcification [30], as well as in those who have had repeated high-energy cardioversions [26]. Other conditions causing myocardial necrosis produce scintigraphic patterns that cannot be distinguished from the patterns resulting from the necrosis due to acute infarction. Thus, patients with myocardial contusion [27] and carcinoma metastatic to the heart show abnormal scintigraphic patterns characteristic of acute infarction.

Since pyrophosphate is a bone-seeker, increased uptake may be seen in overlying ribs in regions of focal pathology. This may occur, for example, in patients with rib fractures due to recent vigorous cardiac massage. Rib uptake can be differentiated from myocardial uptake by demonstrating that the increased activity remains with the ribs rather than the myocardium in multiple projections. A more troublesome problem is increased uptake by calcified costochondral cartilage, which is seen in 1% of patients; in such cases, the interpretation of underlying myocardial activity is hazardous without computer processing. Uptake in calcified skin lesions [32] and breast tumors [28] can be differentiated from myocardial activity by triangulation.

While the diagnostic significance of myocardial scintigraphy with ^{99m}Tc-pyrophosphate is at times unclear, the scintigraphic pattern of myocardial uptake provides clues to the patient's future course, both in hospital and long term [14]. Patients with normal scintigrams have a complication rate of only 5%, both in the hospital and after discharge. Patients with

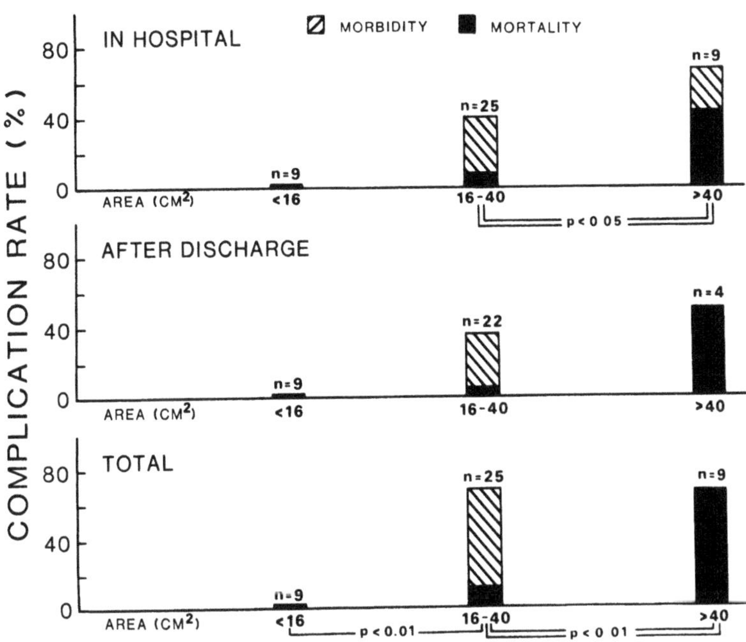

Fig. 3. Complication rates versus area of ^{99m}Tc-pyrophosphate uptake in patients with acute myocardial infarction and focal uptake. (—p<—: complication rate; = p<= : mortality rate.) (Reprinted with permission from [6].)

diffuse uptake and moderate focal uptake (patterns B and C) have a higher morbidity rate than patients with normal scintigrams (total morbidity rates: 36% and 30%, respectively). Patients with pattern D have a high complication rate after discharge (42%). Patients with massive uptake (pattern E) have the highest complication rate of all groups (88% in hospital and 50% after discharge).

If we add additional clinical information, the prognostic information derived from scintigraphy is increased. There is a higher in-hospital complication rate in patients with clinical evidence of acute infarction and focal uptake than in patients without infarction but with similar scintigrams (26% vs. 6%) and in patients with normal scintigrams (26% vs. 5%). The reverse was observed after discharge. While only 6% of patients with acute infarcts and B or C scintigraphic patterns had complications after discharge, 26% of patients without infarction but with abnormal scintigrams had complications after discharge. This may indicate that patients with unstable angina who do not have an infarction during hospitalization continue to have symptoms after discharge until an infarction occurs.

The complication rate, particularly during the hospitalization, is directly related to the extent of the pyrophosphate uptake in patients with acute infarction (Fig. 3). In fact, patients with clinical evidence of infarction and small foci of ^{99m}Tc-pyrophosphate myocardial uptake (less than 16 cm^2) have complication rates comparable to those of patients without acute infarction. On the other hand, when the extent of uptake is moderate (16–40 cm^2), the total complication rate is high (67%). When the extent of uptake is high, the mortality rate is high (87%).

A number of other indices derived from acute infarct scintigraphy appear to have prognostic value. A high incidence of ischemic complications has been observed in patients with focal myocardial uptake of ^{99m}Tc-pyrophosphate persisting for more than six weeks after infarction [21]. Similarly, the incidence of left ventricular failure has correlated well with the extent of ^{99m}Tc-pyrophosphate uptake in patients with acute infarction [41].

There is a good correlation between the size of the acute myocardial infarction and the extent of the scintigraphic abnormality when the infarct is transmural and anterior in location [42–44]. In a canine model, computer-estimated infarct size and gross infarct area correlated well by linear regression analysis ($r=0.95$), as did the computer-estimated in vivo infarct area and the gross infarct area in the right and left anterior oblique projections. The lateral projection showed a poor correlation ($r=0.68$) [43]. These results were corroborated by the findings of another animal study in which good correlation was found between the scintigraphic determinations of infarct area and histologically established infarct weight ($r=0.92$) [42]. While these results suggest that pyrophosphate scintigrams represent a useful, noninvasive method for measuring infarct size, these studies were limited to left anterior descending artery occlusions, and hence the accuracy of estimating diaphragmatic infarct size was not assessed. Other investigators have found a poorer correlation between scintigraphic results and infarct size in inferior wall infarctions [45].

Accurate sizing of the acute infarction by measuring the extent of the radiotracer uptake is limited primarily by the geometric constraints of standard two-dimensional imaging. Single photon emission computed tomography provides a three-dimensional map of radionuclide distribution and may yield more accurate assessments of infarct size. Initial studies in the animal model demonstrated a good correlation ($r=0.85$) between infarct size and measured uptake of ^{99m}Tc-pyrophosphate [45].

Myocardial scintigraphy with ^{99m}Tc-pyrophosphate is useful in patients with suspected acute infarction in whom other clinical and laboratory evidence is nondiagnostic. A negative scintigram is most useful, particularly if it occurs between one and six days after onset of symptoms, since the probability that the patient has had an acute infarction is markedly reduced, and the likelihood of complications is therefore, quite low. The probability that there has been an acute infarction is high in patients with focal uptake, provided they did not have a recent infarct preceding their acute event. The size and persistence of uptake may provide predictive information as well. The usefulness of the test in the face of diffuse uptake is limited, however.

Myocardial scintigraphy can also be used to diagnose right ventricular infarction. While a disproportionate elevation in right ventricular filling pressure may indicate right ventricular involvement, it may also occur in the presence of cor pulmonale. Myocardial scintigraphy with ^{99m}Tc-pyrophosphate provides more direct evidence of acute right ventricular infarction. Sharpe et al. observed right ventricular involvement in six of 15 patients with inferior infarction [47]; five of these patients had right ventricular functional abnormalities including elevated right ventricular filling pressure and right ventricular dilatation or wall motion abnormalities.

This technique is also of value in evaluating patients following cardiac surgery. The diagnosis of myocardial infarction following cardiac surgery is complicated because chest pain, enzyme elevation, and electrocardiographic changes may result from the operation itself [48]. Of 48 patients undergoing coronary artery revascularization surgery [49], six patients (12%) had electrocardiographic evidence of new infarction. All these patients had abnormal scans, but an additional nine patients (total of 15 patients, 31%) had scintigraphic evidence of acute myocardial infarction. When scintigraphy is used for this purpose, it is important that a preoperative scintigram be available for comparison because a significant number of patients going to bypass surgery will have positive infarct scintigrams preoperatively.

Extension or reinfarction can be determined if a baseline scintigram is available. It has been observed, for example, that the abnormalities on infarct scintigraphy may become more prominent during the first 24 to 48 hours after onset of symptoms, even in the absence of clinically suspected infarct extension [20]. On serial infarct scintigrams, certain sequential abnormalities are suggestive of infarct extension: if there is a marked increase in the size of the scintigraphic abnormality shown during the baseline examination, reappearance of an abnormality that had cleared, or appearance of a regional abnormality in an area that was previously normal, reinfarction is likely.

New Infarct-Avid Agents

Other radiotracers have also been used for acute infarct scintigraphy. Accumulation of ^{99m}Tc-glucoheptonate within the infarcted focus has been observed in a number of animal models [50]. Following acute myocardial infarction in the dog, concentration ratios between infarcted and normal myocardium have ranged from 11:1 to 20:1.

The accuracy of this radiotracer in the detection of acute infarction in man appears to be related to the age and size of the infarct. Rossman et al. found that while 80% of all infarcts were detected, moderate and large transmural infarcts could be detected consistently but small subendocardial infarcts could not [51]. In patients with infarcts ranging in age from two to six days, only three of 13 infarcts were detected by scintigraphy [6]. Thus, while this radiotracer may be useful during the early stage of acute infarction, it is not as sensitive as ^{99m}Tc-pyrophosphate after the first day.

Purified radiolabeled antibody against cardiac myosin has also been demonstrated in regions of acute infarction. After the intravenous injection of radioiodine-labeled $(Fab')_2$ fragments of antibodies specific for cardiac myosin, ratios of 6.1 ± 0.6 and 3.3 ± 0.4 between infarcted and normal myocardium have been obtained in the epicardium and endocardium, respectively. There was an inverse relationship between regional myocardial blood flow and uptake of the tracer ($r=-0.81$) [52]. Well-defined areas of increased myocardial activity were detected 72 hours after permanent occlusion of coronary arteries in dogs. Unfortunately, the concentration of tracer within the infarct was too low to permit external detection of the infarct within the first 24 hours after coronary occlusion. The delay in infarct visualization was due to the tracer's prolonged clearance time from the blood and slow entry into the infarct.

A large number of radiopharmaceuticals are sequestered by acutely damaged myocardium. Of the commonly available radiopharmaceuticals, the bone agents, including ^{99m}Tc-pyrophosphate, ^{99m}Tc-diphosphonate, and ^{99m}Tc-methylene diphosphonate, have the highest infarct-to-normal myocardium concentration ratios. Of these, the percent injected dose taken up per gram of damaged tissue is highest with ^{99m}Tc-pyrophosphate. ^{99m}Tc-glucoheptonate and ^{99m}Tc-tetracycline have concentration ratios approximately one half to two thirds that of the bone-seeking tracers. A mercury-containing compound, diiodohydroxymercurifluorescein, yields a concentration ratio between damaged and normal myocardium higher than that of any other radiopharmaceutical tested. In addition, the percent of the injected dose that is taken up per gram of damaged tissue is almost six times that of the bone-seeking radiotracers.

Thus, it appears that structural features can be predicted that will augment the specificity of a radiopharmaceutical for acutely infarcted myocardium. Based on structure:activity relationships such as the presence of mercury and configuration of the organic carrier, it should be possible to synthesize compounds with improved biologic and physical properties for the estimation of acute myocardial infarct size.

References

1. Holman, B.L., Eldh, P., Adams, D.F., Han, M.H., Poggenburg, J.K., Adelstein, S.J.: Evaluation of myocardial perfusion after intracoronary injection of radiopotassium. J. Nucl. Med. 14:274–278 1973
2. Evans, J.R., Gunton, R.W., Baker, R.G., Beanlands, D.S., Spears, J.C.: Use of radioiodinated fatty acid for photoscans of the heart. Circ. Res. 16:1–10 1965
3. Strauss, H.W., Zaret, B.L., Martin, N.D., Wells, H.P., Jr., Flamm, M.D., Jr.: Noninvasive evaluation of regional myocardial perfusion with potassium 43. Technique in patients with exercise-induced transient myocardial ischemia. Radiology 108:85–90, 1973
4. Holman, B.L., Dewanjee, M.K., Idoine, J., Fliegel, C.P., Davis, M.A., Treves, S., Eldh, P.: Detection and localization of experimental myocardial infarction with ^{99m}Tc-tetracycline. J. Nucl. Med. 14:595–599, 1973
5. Holman, B.L., Lesch, M., Zweiman, F.G., Temte, J., Lown, B., Gorlin, R.: Detection and sizing of acute myocardial infarcts with ^{99m}Tc(Sn)tetracycline. N. Engl. J. Med. 291:159–163, 1974
6. Holman, B.L., Tanaka, T.T., Lesch, M.: Evaluation of radiopharmaceuticals for the detection of acute myocardial infarction in man. Radiology 121:427–430, 1976
7. Parkey, R.W., Bonte, F.J., Meyer, S.L., Atkins, J.M., Curry, G.L., Stokely, E.M., Willerson, J.T.: A new method for radionuclide imaging of acute myocardial infarction in humans. Circulation 50:540–546, 1974
8. Bonte, F.J., Parkey, R.W., Graham, K.D., Moore, J., Stokely, E.M.: A new method for radionuclide imaging of myocardial infarcts. Radiology 110:473–474, 1974
9. Zaret, B.L., DiCola, V.C. Donabedian, R.K., Puri, S., Wolfson, S., Freedman, G.S., Cohen, L.S.: Dual radionuclide study of myocardial infarction. Relationships between myocardial uptake of potassium-43, technetium-99m stannous pyrophosphate, regional myocardial blood flow and creatine phosphokinase depletion. Circulation 53:422–428, 1976
10. Shen, A.C., Jennings, R.B.: Myocardial calcium and magnesium in acute ischemic injury. Am. J. Pathol. 67:417–440, 1972
11. Buja, L.M., Tofe, A.J., Mukherjee, A., Parkey, R.W., Bonte, F.J., Willerson, J.T.: Role of elevated tissue calcium in myocardial infarct scintigraphy with technetium phosphorous radiopharmaceuticals. Circulation (Suppl.) 54:II–219, 1976
12. Dewanjee, M.K.: Localization of skeletal-imaging ^{99m}Tc chelates in dead cells in tissue culture: Concise communication. J. Nucl. Med. 17:993–997, 1976
13. Schelbert, H., Ingwall, J., Sybers, H., Ashburn, W: Uptake of Tc-99m pyrophosphate and calcium in irreversibly damaged myocardium. J. Nucl. Med. 17:534, 1976
14. Holman, B.L., Chisholm, R.J., Braunwald, E.: The prognostic implications of acute myocardial infarct scintigraphy with ^{99m}Tc-pyrophosphate. Circulation 57:320–326, 1978
15. Parkey, R.W., Bonte, F.J., Stockely, E.M., Meyer, A.L., Willerson, J.T.: Analysis of Tc-99m stannous pyrophosphate myocardial scintigrams in 242 patients. J. Nucl. Med. 16:556, 1975
16. Ennis, J.T., Walsh, M.J., Mahon, J.M.: Value of infarct-specific isotope (^{99m}Tc-labelled stannous pyrophosphate) in myocardial scanning. Br. Med. J. 3:517–520, 1975
17. Karunaratne, H.B., Walsh, W.F., Fill, H.R., Resnekov, L., Harper, P.V.: Technetium-99m pyrophosphate myocardial scintigraphy in patients with chest pain – lack of diagnostic specificity. J. Nucl. Med. 17:523–524, 1976
18. Cowley, M.J., Mantle, J.A., Rogers, W.J., Russell, R.O. Jr., Rackley, C.E., Logic, J.R.: Technetium-99m stannous pyrophosphate myocardial scintigraphy. Reliability and limitations in assessment of acute myocardial infarction. Circulation 56:192–198, 1977
19. Walsh, W.F., Karunaratne, H.B., Resnekov, L., Fill, H.R., Harper, P.V.: Assessment of diagnostic value of technetium-99m pyrophosphate myocardial scintigraphy in 80 patients with possible acute myocardial infarction. Br. Heart J. 39:974–981, 1977
20. Holman, B.L., Lesch, M., Alpert, J.S.: Myocardial scintigraphy with technetium-99m pyrophosphate during the early phase of acute infarction. Am. J. Cardiol. 41:39–42, 1978
21. Olson, H.G., Lyons, K.P., Aronow, W.S., Brown, W.T., Greenfield, R.S.: Follow-up technetium-99m stannous pyrophosphate myocardial scintigrams after acute myocardial infarction. Circulation 56:181–187, 1977
22. Buja, L.M., Poliner, L.R., Parkey, R.W., Pulido, J.I., Hutcheson, D., Platt, M.R., Mills, L.J., Bonte, F.J., Willerson, J.T.: Clincopathologic study of persistently positive technetium-99m stannous pyrophosphate myocardial scintigrams and myocytolytic degeneration after myocardial infarction. Circulation 56:1016–1023, 1977
23. Ahmad, M., Dubiel, J., Verdon, T.A., Martin, R.H.: Technetium-99m stannous pyrophosphate myocardial imaging in patients with left ventricular aneurysm. Clin. Res. 23:168a, 1975
24. Walsh, W., Lessem, J., Fill, H., Harper, P.V.: Value of ^{99m}Tc-pyrophosphate myocardial scintigraphy in patients with suspected myocardial infarction. Am. J. Cardiol. 37:180. 1976
25. Holman, B.L.: Radionuclide methods in the evaluation of myocardial ischemia and infarction. Circulation (Suppl.) 53:I–112–119, 1976
26. Pugh, B.R., Buja, L.M., Parkey, R.W., Poliner, L.R., Stokely, E.M., Bonte, F.J., Willerson, J.T.: Cardioversion and "false positive" technetium-99m stannous pyrophosphate myocardial scintigrams. Circulation 54:399–403, 1976

27. Go, R.T., Chiu, C.L., Doty, D.B., Cheng, H.F., Christie, J.H.: Radionuclide imaging of experimental myocardial contusion. J. Nucl. Med. 15:1174–1175, 1974
28. Serafini, A.N., Raskin, M.M., Zand, L.C., Watson, D.D.: Radionuclide breast scanning in carcioma of the breast. J. Nucl. Med. 15:1149–1152, 1974
29. Chacko, A.K., Gordon, D.H., Bennett, J.M., O'Mara, R.E., Wilson, G.A.: Myocardial imaging with Tc-99m pyrophosphate in patients on adriamycin treatment for neoplasia. J. Nucl. Med. 18:680–683, 1977
30. Klein, M.S., Coleman, R.E., Roberts, R., Weiss, A.N.: ^{99m}Tc(Sn)pyrophosphate scintigrams in exercise-induced angina and calcified valves. Am. J. Cardiol. 37:149, 1976
31. Jengo, J.A., Mena, I., Joe, S.H., Criley, J.M.: The significance of calcific valvular heart disease in Tc-99m pyrophosphate myocardial infarction scanning: Radiographic, scintigraphic, and pathological correlation. J. Nucl. Med. 18:776–780, 1977
32. Bossuyt, A., Verbeelen, D.: Accumulation of ^{99m}Tc pyrophosphate in the skin lesions of pseudoxanthoma elasticum. Clin. Nucl. Med. 1:245, 1976
33. Hisada, K., Suzuki, Y., Iimori, M.: Technetium-99m pyrophosphate bone imaging in the evaluation of trauma. Clin. Nucl. Med. 1:18–25, 1976
34. Rosenthall, L., Hill, R.O., Chuang, S.: Observation on the use of ^{99m}Tc-phosphate imaging in peripheral bone trauma. Radiology 119:637, 1976
35. Kim, E.: Calcified costal cartilage as a cause of false interpretation on myocardial imaging. Clin. Nucl. Med. 1:159–161, 1976
36. Klein, M.S., Coleman, R.E., Roberts, R., Weiss, A.N.: False positive ^{99m}Tc(Sn)pyrophosphate myocardial infarct images related to delayed blood pool clearance. Clin. Nucl. Med. 1:45–47, 1976
37. Prasquier, R., Taradash, M.R., Botvinick, E.H., Shames, D.M., Parmley, W.W.: The specificity of the diffuse pattern of cardiac uptake in myocardial infarction imaging with technetium-99m stannous pyrophosphate. Circulation 55:61–66, 1977
38. Donsky, M.S., Curry, G.C., Parkey, R.W., Meyer, S.L., Bonte, F.J., Platt, M.R., Willerson, J.T.: Unstable angina pectoris. Clinical, angiographic, and myocardial scintigraphic observations. Br. Heart J. 38:257–263, 1976
39. Abdulla, A.M., Canedo, M.I., Cortez, B.C., McGinnis, K.D., Wilhelm, S.K.: Detection of unstable angina by ^{99m}technetium pyrophosphate myocardial scintigraphy. Chest 69:168–173, 1976
40. Perez, L.A., Hayt, D.B., Freeman, L.M.: Localization of myocardial disorders other than infarction with ^{99m}Tc-labeled phosphate agents. J. Nucl. Med. 17:241–246, 1976
41. Willerson, J.T., Parkey, R.W., Buja, L.M., Harris, R.A., Jr., Stokely, E.M., Blomqvist, G., Bonte, F.J.: Sizing acute myocardial infarction utilizing technetium stannous pyrophosphate myocardial scintigrams in dogs and man. Circulation 52 (Suppl.) 52:I–108, 1975
42. Stokely, E.M., Buja, L.M., Lewis, S.E., Parkey, R.W., Bonte, F.J., Harris, R.A., Jr., Willerson, J.T.: Measurement of acute myocardial infarcts in dogs with ^{99m}Tc-stannous pyrophosphate scintigrams. J. Nucl. Med. 17:1–5, 1976
43. Botvinick, E.H., Shames, D., Lappin, H., Tyberg, J.V., Townsend, R., Parmely, W.W.: Noninvasive quantitation of myocardial infarction with technetium-99m pyrophosphate. Circulation 52:909–915, 1975
44. Holman, B.L., Ehrie, M., Lesch, M.: Correlation of acute myocardial infarct scintigraphy with postmortem studies. Am. J. Cardiol. 37:311–313, 1976
45. Henning, H., Schelbert, H., O'Rourke, R.A., Righetti, A., Hardarson, T., Ashburn, W.: Dual myocardial imaging with Tc-99m pyrophosphate and thallium-201 for diagnosing and sizing acute myocardial infarction. J. Nucl. Med. 17:524, 1976
46. Keyes, J.W., Leonard, P.F., Brody, S.L., Svetkoff, D.J., Rogers, W.L., Lucchesi, B.R.: Myocardial infarct quantification in the dog by single photon emission computed tomography. Circulation 58:227–232, 1978
47. Sharpe, D.N., Botvinick, E.H., Shames, D.M., Schiller, N.B., Massie, B.M., Chatterjee, K., Parmley, W.W.: The noninvasive diagnosis of right ventricular infarction. Circulation 57:483–490, 1978
48. Righetti, A., O'Rourke, R.A., Schelbert, H., Henning, H., Hardarson, T., Daily, P.O., Ashburn, W., Ross, J., Jr.: Usefulness of preoperative and postoperative Tc-99m(Sn)pyrophosphate scans in patients with ischemic and valvular heart disease. Am. J. Cardiol. 39:43–49, 1977
49. Platt, M.R., Parkey, R.W., Willerson, J.T., Bonte, F.J., Shapiro, W., Sugg, W.L.: Technetium stannous pyrophosphate myocardial scintigrams in the recognition of myocardial infarction in patients undergoing coronary artery revascularization. Ann. Thorac. Surg. 21:311–317, 1976
50. Fink-Bennett, D., Dworkin, H.J., Lee, Y.H.: Myocardial imaging of the acute infarct. Radiology 113:449–450, 1974
51. Rossman, D.J., Rouleau, J., Strauss, H.W., Pitt, B.: Detection and size estimation of acute myocardial infarction using ^{99m}Tc-glucoheptonate. J. Nucl. Med. 16:980–985, 1975
52. Khaw, B.A., Beller, G.A., Haber, E.: Experimental myocardial infarct imaging following intravenous administration of iodine-131 labeled antibody $(Fab')_2$ fragments specific for cardiac myosin. Circulation 57:743–750, 1978
53. Davis, M.A., Holman, B.L., Carmel, A.N.: Evaluation of radiopharmaceuticals sequestered by acutely damaged myocardium. J. Nucl. Med. 17:911–917, 1976

Quantitative Assessment of Thallium-201 Images

U. Buell, E. Kleinhans, M. Seiderer, and B.E. Strauer

Radiologische Klinik und Poliklinik der Universität München, Medizinische Klinik I der Universität München, Klinikum Grosshadern, München, FRG

The sensitivity and specificity of thallium-201 myocardial imaging for analysis of regional myocardial viability depends on reproducible image construction and interpretation. Reproducibility is influenced by the myocardial ^{201}Tl uptake, which depends on myocardial perfusion, mass, and metabolism [25, 26]; these factors also determine the myocardial-to-background ratio [7, 14, 15]. Uptake is, in addition, affected by exercise techniques [22], dosage and type of cardiac pharmaceuticals [7, 13, 15, 26], technical equipment, and the methods used for data collection, processing, and display [16]. Accurate interpretation is often difficult, even for experienced investigators. To overcome this problem two techniques are employed: (1) grading analogue images by quality (poor, adequate, or excellent) and by uptake (normal, borderline, or abnormal) [27], and (2) grading of digital images with computer assistance [3–11, 13–18, 20–22].

The accuracy of both methods basically depends on the same factor, i.e., the contrast achieved in the nuclear images. Differences in count rate density and density ratios are used either visually or by the computer to evaluate ^{201}Tl myocardial images. Visual interpretation of unprocessed images led to 67% agreement among four experienced observers in rating the images as either normal, borderline, or abnormal [27]. This evaluation scheme, however, cannot be used to obtain the data on global or regional left ventricular ^{201}Tl uptake, paracardiac or pericardiac count rates, or mediastinal uptake, which are necessary: (1) for correlation with various invasively measured parameters, and (2) for interpretation of ^{201}Tl images of the left ventricle from maximal, minimal, and mean left ventricular ^{201}Tl uptake values. It is the aim of this review to illustrate the various techniques of quantitation of ^{201}Tl images and to discuss treatment of background radioactivity and problems of digital imaging.

Address reprint requests to: Prof. Dr. U. Buell, Radiologische Klinik der Universität München, Klinikum Großhadern, Marchioninistr. 15, D-8000 München 70, Federal Republic of Germany

Technical Needs for Quantitation

While some authors have employed converging collimators for ^{201}Tl left ventricular imaging [9, 11, 14, 18], for quantitation, we recommend a parallel-hole collimator designed for medium resolution and sensitivity. Converging collimators distort the image so that magnification increases with increasing distance from the collimator plane. Nishiyama et al. found that the converging collimator performed poorly with regard to lesion detection [24]. On the other hand, a specially designed seven-pinhole collimator, combined with a computer program, resulted in satisfactory multiplanar emission tomography of the left ventricle [28].

Electrocardiographic gating, which improves spatial resolution by excluding blurring of contours caused by physiologic motion, has been suggested [1, 8, 16]. Gated images acquired over 20 to 30 minutes still, however, have low signal-to-noise ratios. Thallium-201 cinematic imaging with multiple gating [1] seems to be a more promising approach.

Little equipment is needed for quantification, other than what is necessary for obtaining high-quality analogue images. A small, dedicated nuclear medicine computer system routinely includes a core memory permitting use of a 64×64 matrix, background cutoff, and a display-device (television-type video display or oscilloscope display or printer/plotter). If the gamma camera is automatically corrected for uniformity, storage of a correction image is unnecessary. Storage media (tape or disk) are helpful and are necessary if software routines are used for treatment and analysis of digitally acquired images.

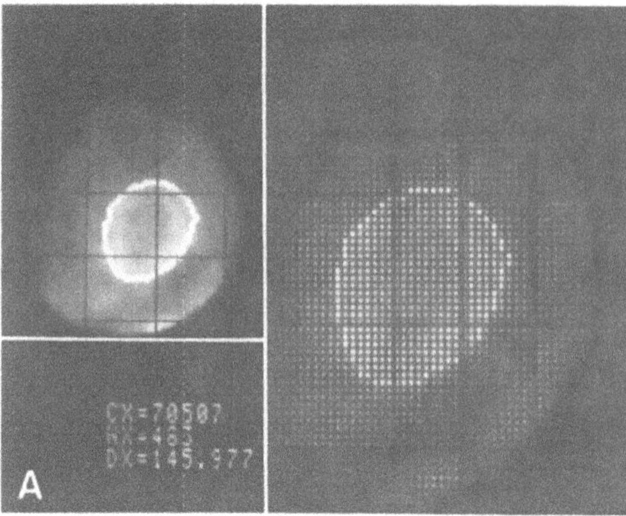

Fig. 1 A and B. Left ventricular hypertrophy in a patient with essential hypertension (45° left anterior oblique projection). **A** Digital image taken from the cathode ray tube display, demonstrating left ventricular ^{201}Tl uptake and distribution (64 × 64 matrix after employment of a magnification factor of 2.5). The pixels included in the left ventricular region of interest are illustrated by magnification on the right. CX denotes counts in the region of interest, NX the number of pixels, and DX the count rate density (CX:NX). **B** Scintimetric plot documenting relative ^{201}Tl uptake in the left ventricular region (see **A**), related to two myocardial maxima (100.0%), using 2 × 2 pixels. Note the homogeneous distribution of 80–99% values in the walls (imaged in tangent) and the valley in the center (66–79% values, anterior wall imaged en face). Q^{201}Tl indicates the left ventricular count rate-to-injected ^{201}Tl dose ratio, and LVMM represents the left ventricular muscle mass.

Computer assistance in ^{201}Tl left ventricular imaging can take two forms: (1) enhancement or treatment of images for better visual analysis [3, 4, 13–18, 20], and (2) statistical analysis of distribution [5–7, 9–11, 21]. If visual evaluation is planned, a 128 × 128 matrix is advantageous [16]. For statistical analysis we prefer the 64 × 64 matrix, "zoomed" by magnification to a 100 × 100 equivalent.

Display Methods

Besides analogue display devices like Polaroid, photographic and x-ray films, digital images can be documented by taking pictures from the computer-processed cathode-ray tube (Fig. 1 A) or video display (Fig. 2). A graded scale can be used to code information in shades of gray or in colors; isodose plots can also be constructed with colors, symbols (Fig. 3 A and B), or contour lines. Scales comprise 10 10% increments (Fig. 3) up to 18 different coded steps (6% increments from 0–100%) [20]. The image contrast can be improved by setting a threshold with cutoff values. In our laboratory, we use a 16-symbol isodose-plotter with a 30% cutoff (from the left ventricular maximum) for printing out ^{201}Tl images. Thus, two symbols for 0–30% and for values exceeding the myocardial maximum excluded, the information is displayed in 5% steps (100% = myocardial maximum, 14 steps cover 30% to 100% of the left ventricular count rate).

Analysis of Analogue Images

Analogue images can be analyzed either visually [27] or by densitometric measurements of scintigraphic films [19]. The latter method has been used in describing semiquantitatively transient transmural reduction of myocardial ^{201}Tl uptake.

Analysis of Digital Images

The methods employed for digital image analysis can be separated into two groups, one that treats the left ventricle as one organ (yielding global data) and another that considers the left ventricle as a sum of segments or small fractions (regional data). For

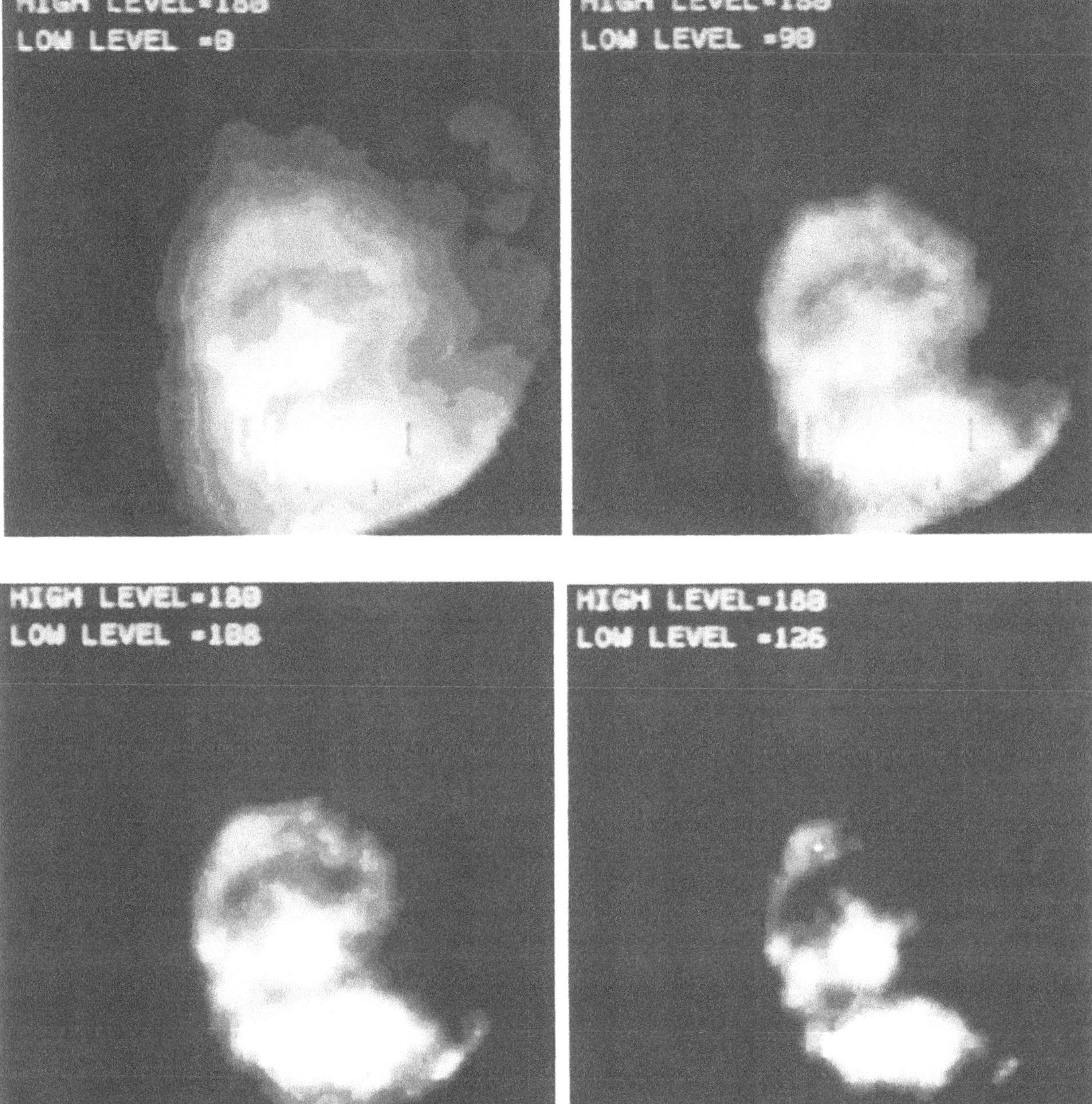

Fig. 2. Left ventricular ^{201}Tl digital images (90° left lateral projection) taken from a computer-processed video display. Cutoff values (percent of myocardial maximum) increase from 0% (top left), to 50% (top right), to 60% (lower left) and to 70% (lower right). Note good visualization of defect contours in the anterior wall in this case of 90% stenosis of the left anterior descending artery. Intestinal ^{201}Tl activity is shown on the bottom.

quantitation, myocardial ^{201}Tl uptake is related to various reference values (Table 1). Thallium-201 activity arising from the myocardium ("net-uptake") is influenced by the left ventricle itself as well as by uptake in the surrounding tissues. Since 50% of the 80 keV emission used for imaging is absorbed by 3.7 cm of water, radiation from the posterior wall in the anteroposterior projection is diminished by the absorption of blood in the left ventricular cavity as well as by the absorption of the anterior wall and the precordial tissues. Moreover, background radiation from lung, blood, and muscle uptake of ^{201}Tl anterior and posterior to the left ventricle is superimposed on the myocardial uptake. This background noise can mask defects in left ventricular myocardial uptake, and subtraction of the background uptake should, therefore, increase the sensitivity of left ventricular ^{201}Tl imaging. Gross and net left ventricular

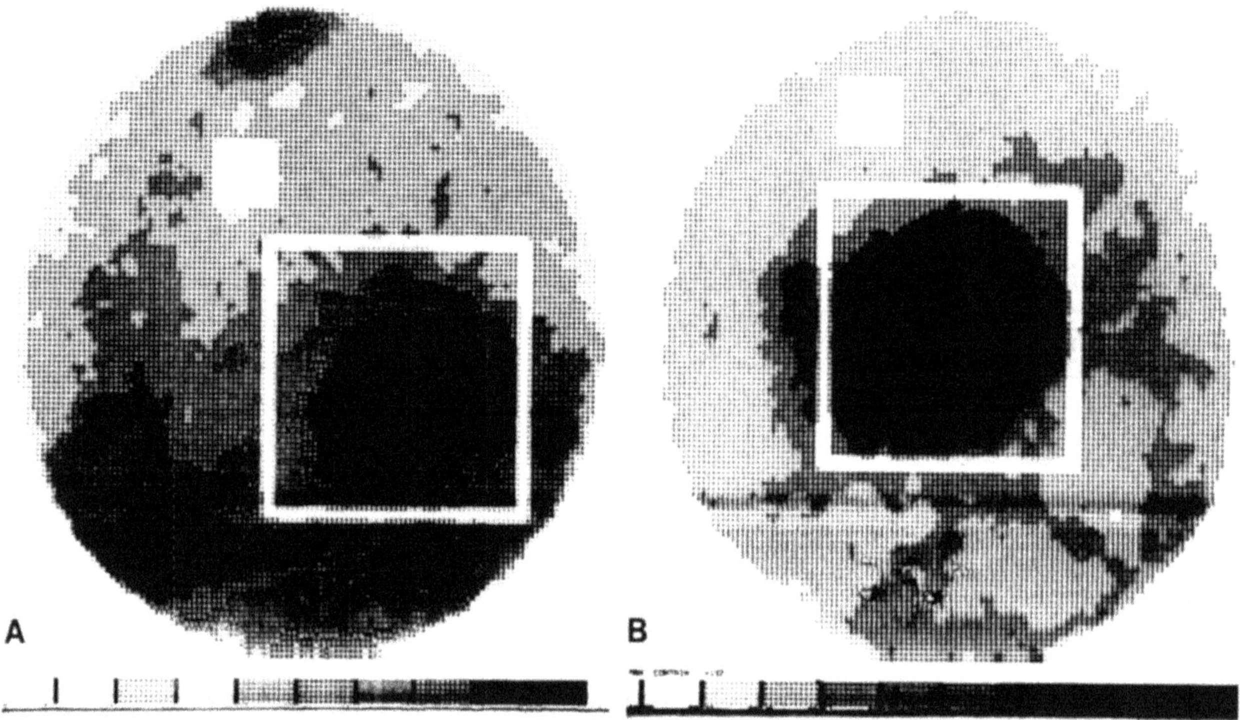

Fig. 3A and B. Isodose plots (10% increments, 45° left anterior oblique projection) of the left ventricle in three-vessel disease at rest (**A**) and after submaximal exercise (**B**). Note the changed distribution after exercise, revealing a new defect at the apex. Paracardiac, mediastinal (square blank region), and myocardial activities and distribution in relation to the myocardial maximum (symbol below on the extreme right) can be determined directly from the image.

Table 1. Reference values for total and regional myocardial ^{201}Tl uptake in patients

Myocardial references
Maximal count rate density [5, 6, 9–11, 16–18, 20, 21]
Count rate density in the left ventricular region
Count rate density opposite the myocardial lesion [3]
Non-myocardial but patient-related references
Paracardiac or lung count rate density [8, 13–15]
Mediastinal count rate density [5, 7]
Liver radioactivity [8]
Count rate density in the thighs [7]
Independent values
Injected dose [7, 13, 26]

Table 2. Background values in left ventricular ^{201}Tl myocardial imaging at rest

1. Experimental determination (dog model) [23]
15–27% of myocardial maximum
(90° left lateral projection, 30 minutes after injection)
2. In man: "paracardiac background" (mean ± SD) [7, 23]
39 ± 9% of myocardial maximum
(45° left anterior oblique projection, 20 minutes after injection)
54 ± 10% of left ventricular count rate density
3. In man: "mediastinal background" (mean ± S.D.)
32 ± 8% of myocardial maximum
(45° left anterior oblique projection, 20 minutes after injection)
34 ± 6% of myocardial maximum
(90° left lateral projection, 26 minutes after injection)
4. Proposed subtraction values [16]
15–25% at rest
10–20% after exercise

^{201}Tl uptake can be computed for both global and regional analysis and related to reference values (Table 1).

Treatment of Background

Background values for in vivo ^{201}Tl myocardial imaging can be derived only from non-background regions such as pericardiac [12, 22], paracardiac [2, 7, 8], and mediastinal [6, 8] areas or from profiles [4]. True background values, determined by Narahara et al. [23] for the 90° left lateral projection in dogs were found to be 15–27% of the myocardial maximum ^{201}Tl uptake (Table 2). Assuming a uniform background, Goris et al. [12] described an interpolative background subtraction: the background was computed by linear interpolation from the count rates found at the edges of a rectangle containing the left

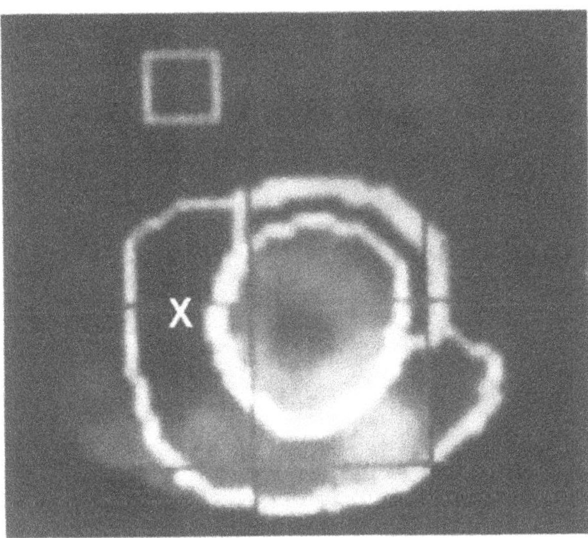

Fig. 4. Regions of interest (45° left anterior oblique projection) used for determining the left ventricular count rate and count rate density (center), as well as the paracardiac (semicircle on top and to the right), and mediastinal (square region) count rate densities. Region x is used for limitation of paracardiac region to areas including the right ventricle and intestine.

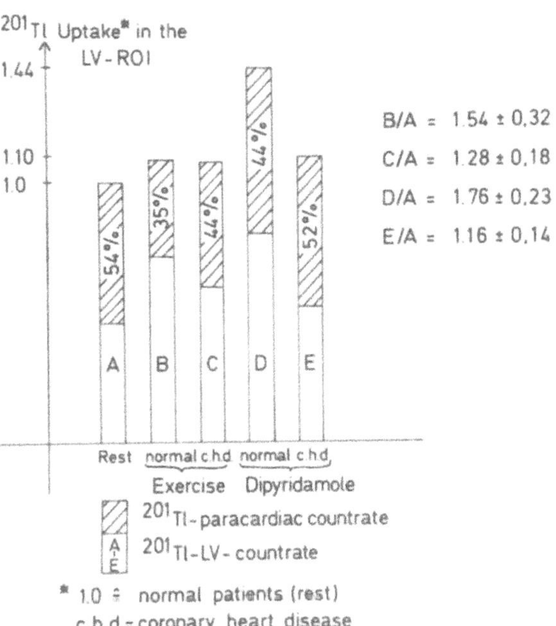

Fig. 5. Portions of paracardiac ^{201}Tl count rate density (background) in absolute values (hatched bars) and as a percentage (%) of total (gross) and net left ventricular count rates (background subtracted; white bars) for the left ventricular region of interest in various conditions. The exercise-to-rest ratios (ordinate: gross; list in upper right: net) show a decrease in absolute and relative paracardiac activity (background) after exercise and the decrease in relative and increase in absolute paracardiac count-rates after dipyridamole. The greatest increase in left ventricular ^{201}Tl uptake (gross: 1.44; net: 1.76) was found in normal individuals.

ventricle. In our laboratory, we have subtracted background values [7] from a paracardiac region, exluding the right ventricle and the intestinal areas; mediastinal uptake was also determined (Fig. 4, Table 2). The paracardiac background was 54% of the left ventricular count rate density, which is roughly equal to a myocardial-to-background ratio of 2:1 [14, 15] and equal to 39% of the maximum left ventricular count rate.

The amount of background interference decreases with increasing time after injection [7] and exercise load (Figs. 3 and 5) and is known to be higher in patients with lung congestion or elevated pulmonary arterial pressure, and after dipyridamole [7]. This causes a wide range of background values among patients. Therefore, for quantitative evaluation of left ventricular ^{201}Tl images, no background subtraction should be performed if inter-individual comparisons are made. Subtraction can be used for intra-individual comparison, for instance in evaluation of rest and exercise uptake in the same patient (Fig. 5), if all other parameters remain unchanged. In these cases and groups, net values of left ventricular ^{201}Tl uptake can be computed from left ventricular count rate densities (mean count rate) (Fig. 5) and from myocardial maximum and minimum count rates as well [7]. Since the real background interference is less than the count rates measured in pericardiac or paracardiac areas, mediastinal ^{201}Tl uptake values (Table 2) would seem to be close to the values proposed by Hamilton et al. for subtraction from rest images [16]. These mediastinal values – representing ^{201}Tl uptake in a sum of non-myocardial tissues – can also be subtracted for correction of images obtained after pharmacologic interventions. On the other hand, it is apparent that background subtraction is an operation that further reduces the already low count rates from the ^{201}Tl uptake in the myocardium. Background cutoff, however, improves detectability of contours without changing the count rates. Therefore, for visual evaluation, cutoff-thresholds can be employed (Fig. 2), sometimes after background subtraction [18].

Evaluation of Global Left Ventricular ^{201}Tl Uptake

The myocardium-to-background ratios derived from the ^{201}Tl myocardial images, which have been used to describe grades of myocardial uptake [8, 13, 15], are equivalent to signal-to-noise ratios. To determine myocardial global ^{201}Tl uptake, a region of interest is drawn containing the left ventricle (Figs. 1, 4, and

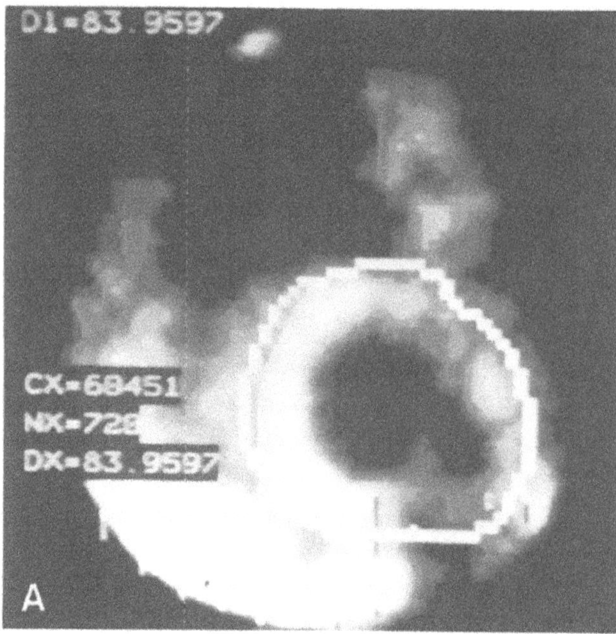

Pat. C.-W. B., 65 J.

präop.

30° LAO

$Q\ ^{201}Tl = 0{,}78$

LVMM ~470 g

$$\frac{Q\ ^{201}Tl}{LVMM} = 1{,}67 \cdot 10^{-3}\,g^{-1}$$

576 688 722 701 670 613 636
663 793 847 878 837 766 755 728 665 574
707 776 858 903 841 770 713 741 716 713 693 559
697 780 847 860 778 691 624 674 676 670 691 668 630
726 770 845 830 707 601 542 567 588 620 670 699 697 649 526
789 812 845 762 611 517 501 515 538 553 620 680 741 762 674
797 830 872 757 582 519 478 480 507 546 601 640 749 787 730 590
780 822 901 778 572 501 494 478 540 559 536 584 707 780 724 578
791 823 881 782 592 505 509 494 513 555 574 580 601 699 728 663 501
797 864 876 745 603 519 526 513 576 613 586 565 622 747 707 665 486
824 899 897 780 649 565 565 597 638 613 594 597 678 726 751 693
951 945 999 889 751 728 716 691 655 645 640 680 747 791 791 553
889 924 985 920 860 797 711 665 636 647 670 701 755 828 668
793 837 887 853 820 720 594 615 647 653 672 697 791
816 734 601 578 567 626 691 645

B

Fig. 6 A and B. Left ventricular aneurysm in coronary heart disease (30° left anterior oblique projection). **A** Left ventricular ^{201}Tl uptake and distribution imaged from a computer-processed video display. Note defects in the anterior wall and in the apex. **B** Scintimetric plot, documenting relative ^{201}Tl uptake in the left ventricular region (see **A**), related to myocardial maximum (99.9%). A defect in the apex is illustrated by uptake value of 59.4% (imaged in tangent). The valley in the center (imaged en face) includes the lowest value in this plot (47.8%), which is significantly below normal. (For explanation of abbreviations see Figure 1.)

6). This procedure raises the problem of accurately determining left ventricular contours; profile techniques or isocount levels have been employed for this, but for such inherently low target/nontarget ratios, the problem has not as yet been solved. Therefore, evaluation methods using the left ventricular circumference as an important parameter in separating normal from abnormal images in inter-individual comparisons [3] could be problematic. This is also true for techniques that measure the number of matrix elements (pixels) imaging the left ventricular walls by defining the left ventricular cavity and myocardial borders [11]. Left ventricular count rate and left ventricular count rate densities are not greatly influenced by this problem and can be used for various correlations.

The ratio of the myocardial (plus precordial) count rate to the injected ^{201}Tl dose in man with the left anterior oblique projection used for imaging 20 minutes after injection of ^{201}Tl – Q ^{201}Tl (Figs. 1 B and 6 B) – correlates well with independent measures of left ventricular muscle mass [26]. Q^{201}Tl may change from laboratory to laboratory since it is based on individual gamma camera and probe sensitivities, the latter used for measuring the syringe containing the injected ^{201}Tl dose. These sensitivities can be kept constant by standard cesium-137 calibrators and/or by multichannel analyzer control.

In a left ventricular ^{201}Tl image, obtained in the 45° left anterior oblique projection from a patient with left ventricular hypertrophy in essential hypertension (Fig. 1 A), the Q^{201}Tl was 1.53 (Fig. 1 B). In contrast, a left ventricular ^{201}Tl image, obtained in the 30° left anterior oblique projection from a patient with a left ventricular aneurysm (Fig. 6 A), showed a Q^{201}Tl of 0.78 (Fig. 6 B). Since the correlation of Q^{201}Tl with the left ventricular muscle mass is linear and the correlation coefficient is 0.89 [26], the portion of viable myocardium in the aneurysmatic left ventricle was about half the left ventricular muscle mass of the patient with hypertrophy. Thus, viable left ventricular muscle mass can be assessed in terms of mass or as a percentage of a standardized value from Q^{201}Tl.

Left ventricular ^{201}Tl count rate densities, computed by division of the left ventricular count rate by the number of pixels included in the region of interest (Figs. 1 A and 6 A) represent mean values of left ventricular ^{201}Tl uptake related to the left ventricular silhouette. Since the dimension of this region of interest, the left ventricular size, is not correlated with the left ventricular muscle mass or any other parameter that determines the left ventricular ^{201}Tl uptake, and since the count rate increases with increase of injected dose, the count rate density is a variable that is of interest only if it is related to a non-myocardial reference in the same patient or to a myocardial reference in the same patient after injection of the same ^{201}Tl dose. In the latter case, background subtraction can be performed for the entire left ventricle with respect to the constant number of pixels included in the left ventricular region of interest. Thus, count rate density values can be compared as net values under varied conditions (rest/exercise, rest/dipyridamole). Dipyridamole-to-rest ratios were successfully correlated with coronary vascular reserve and increase in myocardial oxygen consumption [26]. Exercise-to-rest ratios without background subtraction in normal individuals were found to be approximately 1.0 (1.09 ± 0.12 [7]; 0.92 ± 0.16 [13]). The left ventricular ^{201}Tl net uptake ratio was 1.54 ± 0.32 (Fig. 5; all values mean $\pm$ SD). This difference indicates that the decrease in background radioactivity during exercise masks an increase in left ventricular ^{201}Tl radioactivity. Thus, evaluation of global left ventricular ^{201}Tl uptake revealed pertinent facts concerning the determinants of myocardial ^{201}Tl accumulation and its changes.

Evaluation of Regional Left Ventricular ^{201}Tl Uptake and Distribution

Regional evaluation can be performed using special image enhancement techniques (see above), either visually [8, 22], visually with computer assistance [3, 4, 13–18, 20, 22], or by statistical analysis [5–7, 9–11, 21]. Both profile patterns and color displays are used for evaluation.

Profile Analysis

A profile can be generated over the area of suspected abnormality. The corresponding profile amplitudes then represent regional count rates (or count rate densities) in the slice investigated. Bodenheimer et al. [4] found this technique advantageous, using slices containing one half of the imaged left ventricle, although Hamilton et al. [16] stated that profile methods were no better than visual inspection of the image.

Segmental or Fractional Analysis

Segments or portions of the left ventricle can be described by referring to anatomically defined left ventricular regions [4, 9, 18, 20–22]. For quantitative evaluation, the left ventricular wall or from two [4] to 14 segments of the left ventricle [9] may be analyzed. ^{201}Tl uptake in these left ventricular fractions is defined as pathologically reduced if count rates are less than a threshold, uniformly set from 75% to 80% of the left ventricular ^{201}Tl uptake maximum [4, 18, 20, 21]. Besides the visual analysis of computer-processed images, arbitrarily size-defined regions of 1 cm^2 [8] or visually defined regions are used, the latter chosen to encompass the area of diminished tracer uptake [3]. In these regions, counts per number of pixels enclosed (count rate densities) or minimal counts for four pixels (regional myocardial minima [5, 6]) are computed and related to various reference values (Table 1).

Histograms can be obtained for additional evaluation of ^{201}Tl uptake and homogeneity in the left ventricular walls or segments from determination of the percentage of total pixels allocated to intervals obtained at steps of 10% or 20% of the maximum value or the number of segments with a given count rate density belonging to each interval [11, 21]. Moreover, regional ^{201}Tl uptake and distribution can be determined by normalizing all pixels to the myocardial segment with the maximal count rate density and generating a computer image, deleting all pixels more than three standard deviations below maximal [10], and thereby describing areas of significantly decreased ^{201}Tl uptake. In our laboratory we have developed a scintimetric method [5] employing the 64×64 matrix. A gamma camera with a wide field of view and center magnification is used for aquisition. The number of pixels included in the left ventricular area is, therefore, increased by factor of 2.5 (magnification factor). In effect, the 64×64 matrix is zoomed to a 100×100 matrix. For scintimetric assessments, the 64×64 matrix is reduced to 32×32 by computing ^{201}Tl uptake values as a count rate density for each group of four pixels included in a region of interest containing the left ventricle (Figs. 1 A and 6 A). Values in all 2×2 pixels are plotted as percentages of the maximal count rate density (Figs. 1 B and 6 B), and therefore represent relative regional left ventricular ^{201}Tl uptake.

Printout of the left ventricular ^{201}Tl images is performed with an isodose plotter, using a computed 128×128 matrix. By visually searching for minimal percentage values in the scintimetric plots (Figs. 1 B and 6 B), one for each anatomically defined area (the left ventricular walls) in each projection (anteroposterior, 45° left anterior oblique, 90° left lateral, and

Table 3. Scintimetrically computed relative ^{201}Tl minimum values (mean ± SD) (%) in the left ventricle for a 90° left lateral projection in normal controls and in patients with left anterior descending artery in relation to anatomically defined areas and to number of pixels (100% = myocardial maximum)

Number of pixels[a]	Anterior wall[b]		Posterior wall[c]	
	Normal controls[d]	LAD stenoses[e]	Normal controls	LAD stenoses
1×1	62.1 ± 1.51 * (*)	46.6 ± 9.90	61.4 ± 2.33 * (*)	55.8 ± 8.10
2×2	73.5 ± 1.86 * (*)	58.4 ± 11.2	73.7 ± 4.43 (*)	70.0 ± 7.20
3×3	82.9 ± 5.03 *	65.7 ± 10.6	78.2 ± 4.24	77.9 ± 7.70

[a] 1×1 = 0.14 cm²; 3×3 = 1.26 cm²

[b] Imaged in tangent, segments no. 1 to 3 in Fig. 9, 90° left lateral projection

[c] Imaged in tangent, segments no. 4 to 6 in Fig. 9, 90° left lateral projection

[d,e] $n = 11$

[e] Patients with stenosis of the left anterior descending branch alone; stenosis greater than 90% of luminal diameter

* $p < 0.025$ (Student's *t*-test: normal values vs. normal values; normal values vs. LAD stenoses).

30° right anterior oblique), and assisted by visual topographic analysis of the isodose plot, the minimum was established for each area in each projection. These minimal percentage values were determined in a group of normal individuals to obtain control values. Of these, the mean minus 2 SD ^{201}Tl uptake values were used as a threshold, statistically separating normal minimal ^{201}Tl uptake in each left ventricular region from decreased uptake (Table 3). Minimum ^{201}Tl uptake values are different for each region ([5] Table 3) or left ventricular segment [9]. These differences become smaller during exercise [6, 7], but the use of uniform values or thresholds [4, 18, 20, 21] for all anatomical areas or segments of the left ventricle viewed in one image remains problematic.

Minimum values can be used not only to classify regional ^{201}Tl uptake as normal or abnormal, but also for correlation with various other parameters [5, 7]. For instance, minimum values were different in normokinesis as compared with dyskinesis or akinesis (Fig. 7). These relations were confirmed by Hamilton et al. [14] and by Bodenheimer et al. [4]. Moreover, mediastinal ^{201}Tl uptake as a percentage of

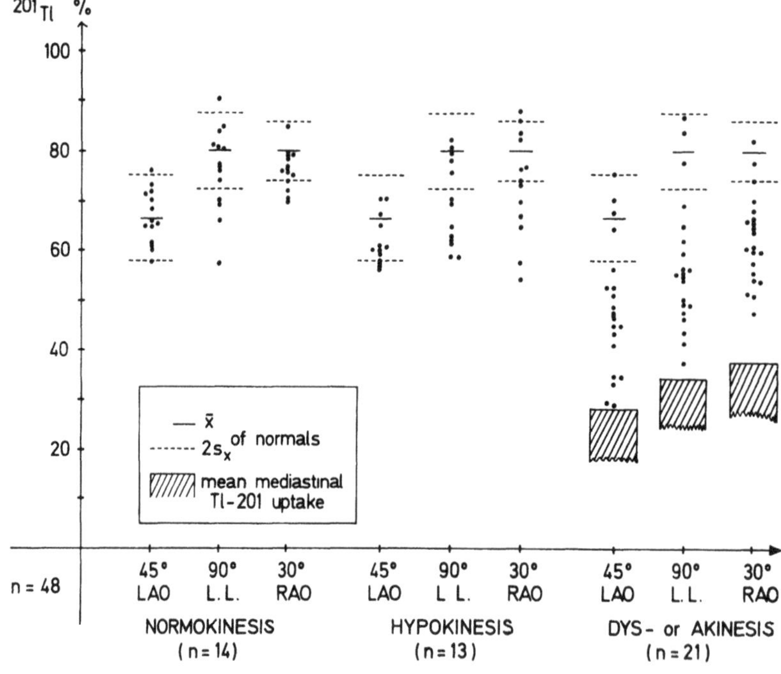

Fig. 7. Relationship between anterior wall motion (cineventriculographically determined) and relative minimal ^{201}Tl uptake in this left ventricular area (imaged in three projections), demonstrated by individual values obtained from patients with coronary heart disease (points) in comparison to the normal controls and to the mediastinal count rate density [5]. Note the decrease of ^{201}Tl uptake with increasing asynergy which reaches lowest values in the group of patients with dyskinesis or akinesis. In the 45° left anterior oblique projection, mediastinal ^{201}Tl uptake can be used as a reference for areas in the anterior wall whose accumulation capacity does not differ from that of mediastinal tissue, and which are, therefore, probably nonviable.

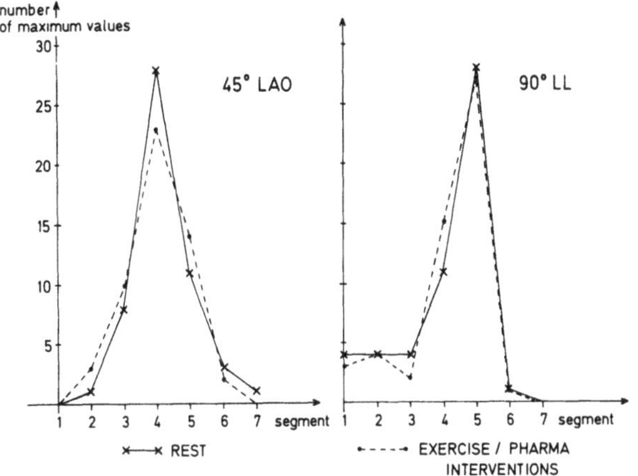

Fig. 8. Segmental location of left ventricular ^{201}Tl maximum uptake in 45° left anterior oblique and in 90° left lateral projections at rest and after exercise and pharmacologic interventions, respectively. (For segment description see Fig. 9.) Note the virtually unchanged location of maximum uptake values in segments no. 4 (45° left anterior oblique projection and no. 5 (90° left lateral projection) in both normal individuals and patients.

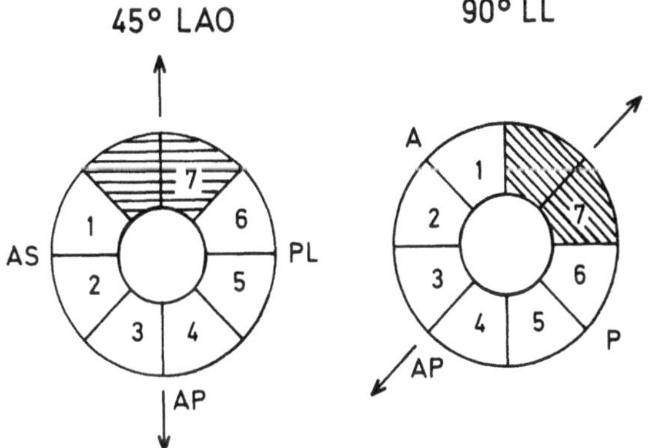

Fig. 9. Subdivisions of myocardium for two projections (45° left anterior oblique, and 90° left lateral) into 7+1 (center) segments each.

the myocardial maximum represents a limit for myocardial uptake in terms of myocardial viability: the closer minimal ^{201}Tl uptake in the left ventricular anterior wall is to the mediastinal one, the more likely the left ventricular area is to be non-viable (Fig. 7). This is especially true for the anterior wall imaged in the left anterior oblique projection, since either area (anterior wall and mediastinal reference) is imaged en face (Fig. 4).

Analysis of Left Ventricular ^{201}Tl Maximal and Minimal Uptake Values

Since the quantitative assessment of left ventricular ^{201}Tl images refers primarily to the myocardial ^{201}Tl uptake maximum (Table 1), the question of whether

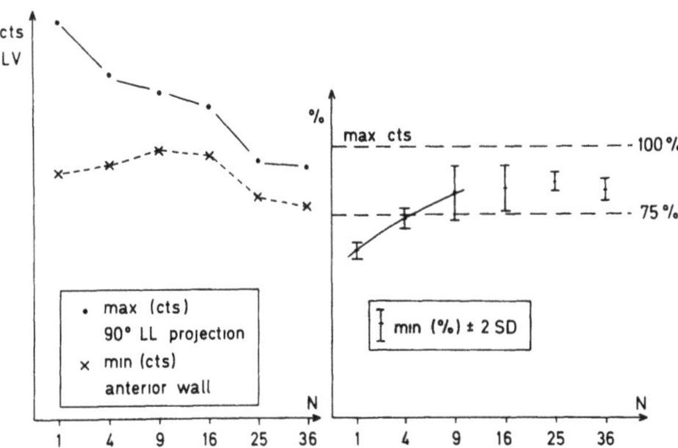

Fig. 10. Count rate densities obtained from the anterior wall (90° left lateral projection) in normal individuals with reference to the number of pixels used for evaluation (1 × 1 to 6 × 6) (left). Note the decrease in maximal count rate density with increasing number of pixels. On the right, the maximal count rate density is assumed to be 100% for all numbers of pixels used, and the minimal count rate density is expressed as a percentage of the maximum. Note the increase in minimal uptake values, which are mathematically correct up to 3 × 3 (9 pixels); 75% cutoff values can be employed from 4 × 4 pixels on. This threshold proved to be too high for 1 × 1 to 3 × 3 pixels, i.e., for 0.14–1.26 cm^2 per region.

this reference is reliable arises. Figure 8 shows that the area of maximum uptake among seven left ventricular segments studied in two projections (Fig. 9), does not vary greatly during exercise or after pharmacologic (dipyridamole, dobutamine) interventions as compared with the location at rest. In the 45° left anterior oblique projection, maximal ^{201}Tl uptake can most likely be expected in segment no. 4 (Fig. 9), which represents an area in the posterolateral wall close to the apex. In the 90° left lateral projection, it is segment no. 5, i.e., the posterior wall. Both areas are imaged in tangent.

In contrast, the maximal count level does not seem to be constant under all conditions. At rest, the maximum uptake value proved to be independent of the type of heart disease [5]. After comparing left ventricular maximum values in the same patients at rest and during exercise, we found that the left ventricular maximum uptake increased by a factor of 1.48 (normal individuals, background subtracted), while thigh uptake increased by a factor of 4.9 [7]. In coronary heart disease, the left ventricular maximum increased by only 1.30, while thigh uptake was increased by 4.63 [7]. Dipyridamole-to-rest ratios were 1.70 (normal individuals, background subtracted) and 1.19 (coronary heart disease patients) (Fig. 5). Thus, maximal left ventricular ^{201}Tl uptake values during exercise and after pharmacologically induced luxury perfusion (with dipyridamole) may not be the constants they should be for reference. After dipyridamole, areas of left ventricular ^{201}Tl maximum uptake in coronary heart disease increased significantly less

($p < 0.005$) in uptake than did areas of maximum uptake in the normal left ventricle. During exercise, most ^{201}Tl accumulates in the stressed skeletal muscles and not in the left ventricle. It is as yet not clear whether maximal left ventricular ^{201}Tl uptake during exercise represents a maximum label in man.

The maximal and minimal ^{201}Tl counts, measured in the anterior wall of the left ventricle (90° left lateral projection), also depend on the number of pixels used for evaluation. Maximal count rate densities, in particular, decrease with increasing number of pixels used for reference (1×1 to 6×6). Thus, if the minimal count rates are expressed as a percentage of the maximal count rates (maximum assumed to be constantly 100%), the differences between these two values decreases with increasing number of pixels. If more than 3×3 pixels are used, minimal values leave the asymptotic curve representing the mathematical model (Fig. 10) because from 4×4 pixels on, these square regions of interest can exceed the myocardial wall, imaged in tangent. Since one pixel is equivalent to $0.14\ cm^2$ in the model presented, 4×4 pixels represent $2.24\ cm^2$ of the left ventricular region of interest. Using 6×6 pixels, i.e., a count rate density of 36 pixels in a square region ($5.04\ cm^2$) seems to be inadequate for regional quantitation.

From these findings it is obvious that a 75% cutoff level can be reasonably employed as a lower limit only if 16 pixels or more are used for quantitatively expressing regional left ventricular ^{201}Tl uptake. Therefore, normal values for relative ^{201}Tl uptake must be computed by taking into account the number of pixels used for the evaluation. From the standard deviations derived from normal values using one pixel only, this matrix seems to be acceptable (Fig. 10, Table 3). On the other hand, determining relative minimal ^{201}Tl uptake in stenoses of the left anterior descending artery (greater than 90% of luminal diameter), similar sensitivities could be obtained by using 2×2 or 3×3 pixels. Moreover, the specificity of values obtained from 1×1 pixels was inferior because of a false-positive decrease ($p < 0.025$) found in the *posterior* wall uptake in patients with stenosis of the left anterior descending artery alone as compared with normal controls. In addition, a pixel size of $0.14\ cm^2$ may be inaccurate for statistical analysis of an organ because of blurring due to motion. This argument must also be considered if image subtraction (exercise minus rest) is performed to illustrate and compute changes in distribution within the left ventricle [16]. We found the statistics of such point-to-point differences too poor for practicable use when a 1×1 pixel was used. For scintimetric evaluation 2×2 pixels ($0.56\ cm^2$) have been used routinely in our laboratory since 1975 [5–7, 26].

Conclusion

Since quantitative assessment of ^{201}Tl images is mainly used as an aid or a complement to visual evaluation, its usefulness may be in assessing questionable findings and in reducing observer bias rather than in establishing new diagnostic criteria. However, it is apparent that results reported from computer-assisted evaluation of left ventricular ^{201}Tl images show higher sensitivity and specificity than findings from simple visual analysis [4, 5, 9, 18]. This cumulates in a 96% sensitivity in detecting coronary heart disease [10]. Moreover, such easily derived values as left ventricular count rate have proved to be informative parameters [7, 13, 15, 26].

The difficulties involved in the use of maximal left ventricular ^{201}Tl uptake values as a reference seem to be decreased by using one ^{201}Tl injection for both rest and exercise imaging ("redistribution analysis") [17], since the diagnosis is not made from absolute but from relative changes within a related distribution image. The problems that remain to be solved for reliable and reproducible employment of quantifying methods are: (1) determination of the correct border of the left ventricular wall (imaged in tangent) with respect to both the left ventricular cavity (imaged posterior to the en-face-viewed myocardium) and to paracardiac activity, and (2) determination of the correct background values to be subtracted. Some of these problems may be resolved by more advanced imaging techniques as, for example, computerized emission tomography.

References

1. Alderson, P.O., Wagner, H.N., Gomez-Moeiras, J.J., Rehn, T.G., Becker, L.C., Douglas, K.H., Manspeaker, H.F., Schindledecker, G.R.: Simultaneous detection of myocardial perfusion and wall motion abnormalities by cinematic ^{201}Tl imaging. Radiology 127:531–533, 1978
2. Atkins, H.L., Budinger, T.F., Lebowitz, E., Ansari, A.N., Greene, M.W., Fairchild, R.G., Ellis, K.J.: Thallium-201 for medical use. Part 3: Human distribution and physical imaging properties. J. Nucl. Med. 18:133–140, 1977
3. Blood, D.K., McCarthy, D.M., Sciacca, R.R., Cannon, P.J.: Comparison of single-dose and double-dose thallium-201 myocardial perfusion scintigraphy for the detection of coronary artery disease and prior myocardial infarction. Circulation 58:777–788, 1978
4. Bodenheimer, M.M., Banke, V.S., Fooshee, C., Hermann, G.A., Helfant, R.H.: Relationship between regional myocardial perfusion and the presence, severity and reversibility of asynergy in patients with coronary heart disease. Circulation 58:789–795, 1978
5. Buell, U., Niendorf, H.P., Strauer, B.E., Hast, B.: Evaluation of myocardial function with the ^{201}thallium scintimetry in various diseases of the heart: A correlative study based on 100 patients. Europ. J. Nucl. Med. 1:125–136, 1976
6. Buell, U., Strauer, B.E., Witte, J.: Segmental analysis of Tl-201 stress myocardial scintigraphy: The problem of using uniform

normal values of Tl-201 myocardial uptake (letter). J. Nucl. Med. 18:1240–1241, 1977
7. Buell, U., Strauer, B.E., Bürger, S., Witte, J., Niendorf, H.P.: Effects of physical stress and pharmacologically induced coronary dilation on myocardial and non-myocardial ^{201}thallium-uptake. Europ. J. Nucl. Med. 3:19–27, 1978
8. Cook, D.J., Bailey, I., Strauss, H.W., Rouleau, J., Wagner, H.N., Jr., Pitt, B.: Thallium-201 for myocardial imaging: Appearance of the normal heart. J. Nucl. Med. 17:583–589, 1976
9. Emrich, D., Rentrop, P., Facorro, L., Karsch, R., Schicha, H., Carstens, B., Kreuzer, H.: Limitations of thallium-201 scintigraphy for evaluation of chronic ischemic heart disease (abstract) World Federation of Nuclear Medicine and Biology: Second International Congress, Washington D.C., Sept. 17–21, 1978, p. 50
10. Faris, J.V., Burt, R.W., Graham, M.C., Knoebel, S.B.: Improved sensitivity in detecting coronary artery disease using computer statistical analysis of thallium-201 scans. World Federation of Nuclear Medicine and Biology: Second International Congress, Washington D.C., Sept. 17–21, 1978, p. 93
11. Fletcher, J.W., Walter, K.E., Witztum, K.F., Daly, J.L., Herbig, F.K., Mueller, H.S., Donati, R.M.: Diagnosis of coronary artery disease with ^{201}Tl: Computer analysis of myocardial perfusion images. Radiology 128:423–427, 1978
12. Goris, M.L., Daspit, S.G., McLaughlin, P., Kriss, J.P.: Interpolative background subtraction. J. Nucl. Med. 17:744–747, 1976
13. Gould, K.L., Westcott, R.J., Albro, P.C., Hamilton, G.W.: Noninvasive assessment of coronary stenoses by myocardial imaging during pharmacologic coronary vasodilation. II. Clinical methodology and feasibility. Am. J. Cardiol. 41:279–287, 1978
14. Hamilton, G.W., Trobaugh, G.B., Ritchie, J.L., Williams, D.L., Weaver, W.D., Gould, K.L.: Myocardial imaging with intravenously injected thallium-201 in patients with suspected coronary artery disease: Analysis of technique and correlation with electrocardiographic, coronary anatomic and ventriculographic findings. Am. J. Cardiol. 39:347–354, 1977
15. Hamilton, G.W., Narahara, K.A., Yee, H., Ritchie, J.L., Williams, D.L., Gould, K.L.: Myocardial imaging with thallium-201: Effect of cardiac drugs on myocardial images and absolute tissue distribution. J. Nucl. Med. 19:10–16, 1978
16. Hamilton, G.W., Ritchie, J.L., Williams, D.L.: Specialized computer aquisition, analysis and display of thallium-201 myocardial images. In: Thallium-201 Myocardial Imaging, edited by J.L. Ritchie, G.W. Hamilton, F.J.Th. Wackers. New York, Raven Press, 1978, pp. 133–150
17. Hör, G., Sebening, H., Sauer, E., Lichte, H., Dressler, J., Lutilsky, L., Wagner-Manslan, C., Pabst, H.W.: Clinical experience with ^{201}Tl-myocardial scintigraphy (redistribution analysis) and ECG-gated blood pool scan. Herz 2:215–216, 1977
18. Lenaers, A., Block, P., Thiel, van E., Lebedelle, M., Becquevort, P., Erbsmann, F., Ermans, A.M.: Segmental analysis of Tl-201 stress myocardial scintigraphy. J. Nucl. Med. 18:509–516, 1977
19. Maseri, A., Parodi, O., Severi, S., Pesola, A.: Transient transmural reduction of myocardial blood flow, demonstrated by thallium-201 scintigraphy, as a cause of variant angina. Circulation 54:280–288, 1976
20. Mathey, D., Montz, R., Hanrath, P., Knop, J., Kupper, W., Schneider, C., Bleifeld, W.: Reversible Myokardischämie oder irreversible Myokardfibrose? Dt. Med. Wochenschr. 103:1736–1739, 1978
21. McKillop, J.H., Bessent, R.G., Murray, R.G., Turner, J.G., Tweddel, A., Greig, W.R.: Quantitative approach to the analysis of the normal thallium-201 myocardial image. Europ. J. Nucl. Med. 3:223–225, 1978
22. McLaughlin, P.R., Martin, R.P., Doherty, P., Daspit, S., Goris, M., Haskell, W., Lewis, S., Kriss, J.P., Harrison, D.C.: Reproducibility of thallium-201 myocardial imaging. Circulation 55:497–503, 1977
23. Narahara, K.A., Hamilton, G.W., Wiliams. D.L., Gould, K.L.: Myocardial imaging with thallium-201: An experimental model for analysis of true myocardial and background image components. J. Nucl. Med. 18:781–786, 1977
24. Nishiyama, H., Romhilt, D.W., Williams, C.C., Adolph, R.J., Sodd, V.J., Blue, J.W., Lewis, J.T., Gabel, M., van der, Bel Kahn, J.M.: Collimator evaluation for Tl-201 myocardial imaging. J. Nucl. Med. 19:1067–1073, 1978
25. Strauer, B.E., Bürger, S., Buell, U.: Multifactoral determination of ^{201}thallium uptake of the heart: an experimental study concerning the influence of ventricular mass, perfusion and oxygen consumption. Basic Res. Cardiol. 73:298–306, 1978
26. Strauer, B.E., Buell, U., Bürger, S.: Clinical studies concerning the determinants of myocardial ^{201}Tl uptake. Basic Res. Cardiol. 73:365–379, 1978
27. Trobaugh, G.B., Wackers, F.J.Th., Sokole, E.B., De Rouen, T.A., Ritchie, J.L., Hamilton, G.W.: Thallium-201 myocardial imaging: An interinstitutional study of observer variability. J. Nucl. Med. 19:359–363, 1978
28. Vogel, R.A., Kirch, D., LeFree, M., Steele, P.: A new method of multiplanar emission tomography using a seven pinhole collimator and an anger scintillation camera. J. Nucl. Med. 19:648–654, 1978

Thallium-201 Myocardial Perfusion Scintigraphy during Rest and Exercise

A. Lenaers

Service de Diagnostic par Radioisotopes, Hôpital Universitaire Saint-Pierre, Brussels, Belgium

In 1973 Zaret and coworkers described a method for the noninvasive visualization of stress-induced myocardial ischemia in patients with coronary artery disease by the intravenous injection of radioactive potassium during both rest and treadmill exercise. In patients with angina pectoris, regions of relatively decreased ^{43}K accumulation were identified when the tracer was administered during exercise but were not found at rest. These zones of relative hypoperfusion corresponded to regions supplied by angiographically demonstrable stenotic coronary arteries in all patients [1]. This method was also applied to the noninvasive evaluation of patients with false-positive exercise tests [2] and after coronary artery bypass surgery [3].

Unfortunately, the gamma-ray spectrum of ^{43}K, with its two main peaks at 373 and 619 keV, includes photon energies that do not allow optimal scintigraphic resolution with the collimators commercially available for gamma cameras, and thus require special shielding by 5-cm-thick lead bricks or the use of rectilinear scanners [4].

The same problem arose with rubidium-81, a potassium analogue, because of its abundant high energy gamma emissions (511 keV) and the contaminant rubidium-82m. Without a special shield, image resolution was inadequate [5]. With special shielding, however, rest and stress ^{81}Rb scintigraphy provided greater sensitivity and specificity when compared to stress electrocardiography in the noninvasive identification of significant coronary stenosis [5, 6] and proved to be useful in the assessment of myocardial perfusion improvement after coronary artery bypass surgery [7].

The use of thallium-201, another potassium analogue, was proposed in 1973 by Lebowitz [8]. This radionuclide decays by electron capture, emits gamma photons of 135 and 167 keV in 10% total abundance and mercury-characteristic x-rays of 69–83 keV in 98% abundance [9]. Its 73-hour half-life gives ^{201}Tl a good shelf life, but the effective whole-body half-time of about 57 hours is a drawback when studies are to be repeated at short intervals [10, 11].

Thallium-201 compares favorably with ^{43}K and ^{81}Rb for myocardial perfusion imaging with currently available equipment [12]. Moreover, its biologic properties make it a good tracer for visualization of transient stress-induced ischemia, since its blood concentration decreases to less than 3% of the injected dose in a few minutes, while the concentration in the heart decreases with a half-time of over seven hours [13].

Basic Considerations

In patients with coronary artery disease, myocardial perfusion scintigraphy with injection of ^{201}Tl at rest allows the detection of myocardial infarction or severe ischemia [14]. Most patients with coronary artery stenoses, however, have normal rest perfusion scintigrams if there are no areas of infarction. As demonstrated by Gould et al. in dogs, the resting flow distal to a stenotic coronary artery may be normal if the lumen is narrowed by less than 85–90% [15]. In contrast, during stress in patients with coronary artery disease, there is a limitation to flow increase, and an inverse relationship between the increase in flow and percent coronary artery stenosis is shown once the lumen is narrowed by approximately 40–50% [16]. Thus, if the initial distribution of thallium reflects the distribution of regional blood flow, injection at peak exercise should allow detection of myocardial stress-induced ischemia in patients with coronary artery disease.

The concentration of ^{201}Tl in the myocardium immediately following injection of the tracer reflects

Address reprint requests to: André Lenaers, M.D., Service de Diagnostic par Radioisotopes, Hôpital Universitaire Saint-Pierre, Rue Haute, 322, B-1000 Brussels, Belgium

both blood flow and the extraction fraction. The latter is defined as the ratio (A–V)/(A), where A and V are the arterial and the venous concentrations, respectively. The extraction fraction has been studied in dogs under various conditions, including changes in heart rate or pH, hypoxia, reactive hyperemia, and injection of adenosine, insulin, strophantidine, or propanolol. A constant value of 88% has been found under most conditions, with only a moderate fall to 78% with hypoxemia or acidosis, and a progressive decrease when myocardial blood flow was increased in excess of demand [17]. The effect of hypoxemia and acidosis on extraction fraction is probably related to their effect on the sodium-potassium adenosine triphosphatase (ATPase) pump system of the myocardial cell membrane [17, 19]. However, when hypoxia results from hypoperfusion, an increased extraction at very low flow rates may compensate for this effect, as has been demonstrated with other potassium analogues [18, 19]. Under conditions of partial coronary occlusion in dogs, the regional uptake of ^{201}Tl closely parallels the distribution of microspheres [20]. Thus, immediately after thallium administration, the regional concentration of tracer in the myocardium may be considered representative of blood flow. When thallium is administered during exercise, imaging should be performed as soon as possible to visualize areas of reduced thallium uptake corresponding to stress-induced ischemia. Pohost et al. have demonstrated that the areas of reduced thallium uptake visualized immediately after exercise progressively disappear in 1–6 hours, except in the regions where the myocardium is irreversibly damaged [21].

Thus, myocardial defects due to transient stress-induced ischemia may be missed if imaging is delayed [21]. In dogs submitted to transient coronary occlusion, this redistribution corresponds to little decrease in ^{201}Tl uptake in normal areas but an important increase in previously ischemic regions [22].

Instrumentation

Good myocardial images may be obtained with rectilinear scanners or scintillation cameras [23]. For stress myocardial scintigraphy, however, all scintigrams must be collected rapidly in order to avoid significant redistribution of the tracer to transient ischemic areas. Only gamma cameras are able to provide scintigrams of acceptable quality in multiple projections within thirty minutes.

The spatial resolution of a gamma camera depends on the photon energy of the radionuclide and the intrinsic resolution of the camera and collimator. Although the 69–83 keV x-rays of ^{201}Tl are near the low end of the scale for resolution, they are detected seven times as frequently as the 135–167 keV gamma photons despite increased absorption of the x-rays by the overlying chest wall [11]. Several collimators have been proposed for ^{201}Tl stress myocardial imaging. Groch and Lewis, using a thyroid phantom and a Pho Gamma HP camera, suggested the use of a low-energy converging rather than a high-resolution collimator [24]. Graham et al. found a very small difference in resolution when comparing a low-energy converging, a medium-energy converging and a pinhole collimator [25], but the sensitivity of the pinhole collimator is too low to allow collection of enough counts before significant redistribution of the tracer. In our own experience, a converging collimator has two advantages: (1) it diminishes the contribution of noncardiac tissues to the image, especially abdominal organs that have significant thallium uptake, like the stomach, and (2) it reduces the counting time by a factor of 0.6 as compared with collimators of similar resolution. If parallel-hole collimators are used, an all-purpose collimator will offer the best compromise between good resolution and good sensitivity. High-resolution collimators are time consuming and are not very useful since the cyclic displacement of the myocardium is about 1–2 cm. It seems preferable to use a collimator that results in a more rapid imaging so that scintigrams in multiple projections can be collected [26]. Even with multiple projections, however, small ischemic zones of less than 1 cm may escape detection. Fortunately, as outlined by Holman, the ischemic vascular beds to be imaged are usually relatively large, since clinically significant obstruction of the coronary arteries usually involves proximal vessels [19].

Exercise Testing

Work loads are now almost exclusively imposed by means of motor-driven treadmills or bicycle ergometers with mechanical or electromagnetic breaking. Treadmills are used mostly in the United States, while bicycles, either with the subject supine or in the upright position, are usually preferred in Europe. Both devices have advantages, and the final choice finally relies on local experience and local population habits.

Both for safety and because of diagnostic requirements, the entire test and recovery sequence should be performed under continuous monitoring with at least three electrocardiograph (ECG) leads. The three most sensitive leads for detection of stress-induced abnormalities are V_2, V_5 and aVF or an equivalent chest lead. If a fourth channel is available, D_1, V_2, V_5, aVF or V_2, V_4, V_6, aVF may be used [27].

For diagnostic purposes, it is recommended that a multistage test with a series of continuously increasing loads be performed [27]. The physician should choose the initial workload according to the patient's age, history, clinical status, and training, and the increment according to the cardiovascular response to the first load. In most cases, 50 W or 75 W are suitable for the first load and 25 W for each incremental increase.

No more than four successive stages should be imposed, as fatigue will become the limiting factor. An almost steady state must be reached at each level. This is of greater importance in the testing of patients with suspected coronary artery disease in order to avoid abrupt overloading of the heart. A duration of 3–5 minutes for each level meets these requirements. The blood pressure and the clinical status of the patient must be regularly checked, at least once at each level, and preferably during the last minute. The test should be continued until at least 90% of the predicted maximal heart rate is achieved, which is the difference between 220 and the patient's age. Two millicuries of ^{201}Tl thallous chloride should then be injected through an intravenous cannula inserted into a cubital vein before the exercise test. The patient should be asked to continue the test at the same load for at least another minute to allow adequate distribution of the tracer. In order to prevent orthostatic hypotension, patients who have been on a bicycle ergometer in the sitting position should continue cycling for one additional minute under little or no load before stopping completely.

Subjective criteria for stopping the test are severe dyspnea, dizziness, or near syncope; significant chest discomfort or pain suggestive of angina pectoris; intense fatigue; and marked claudication [27]. Objective criteria are an abnormal blood pressure response and the appearance of severe ECG changes. The failure of blood pressure to increase and, in particular, a fall in systolic blood pressure or pulse pressure with exertion is an indication for stopping the test. Excessive elevation of systolic blood pressure (250–280 mm Hg) is considered another limiting sign by most cardiologists. Severe ECG changes include the appearance of supraventricular or ventricular paroxysmal tachycardia, ventricular ectopic beats occurring before the end of a T wave, three or more successive ectopic ventricular complexes, increased frequency of ventricular ectopic complexes during exercise, second or third degree atrio-ventricular block, major left intraventricular conduction disturbances, and horizontal or divergent ST-segment displacement of at least 0.2 mV as compared with the resting ECG. These changes suggest that the subject has reached a level beyond which further exertion would provide little additional information and would be poorly tolerated or even hazardous [27]. When the exercise test is stopped before reaching 90% of the predicted maximal heart rate, for any of these limiting symptoms or signs, ^{201}Tl is injected immediately, and the same or a lower load is imposed for one more minute. If ST-segment depression occurs during exercise, ^{201}Tl is injected when the depression reaches 0.1 mV, although exercise is continued as described above.

The stress level is an important factor. When no limiting symptom occurs, 90% of the predicted maximal heart rate must be reached in order to avoid a higher incidence of false-negative scintigrams. Among 150 patients studied by exercise scintigraphy, exercise ECG, and coronary arteriography, we observed no limiting symptoms in 21 cases [28]. A heart rate of at least 90% of maximum was reached in 19 patients. No patient in this group had a false-negative scintigram, while both other subjects did. To assess the effect of varying the level of exercise, McLaughlin et al. submitted 12 patients to light exercise tests in addition to rest and maximum exercise studies and observed that only 53% of ischemic defects present at maximum exercise were seen in the light exercise study [29]. Thus, significant coronary disease can be missed with less than maximum exercise.

Computer Processing

Scintigrams may be recorded on Polaroid film directly from the cathode ray display of the gamma camera or stored in a computer as digitized images, allowing background suppression, contrast enhancement, or quantitation of regional myocardial uptake. Threshold substraction of 10–50% of the maximum activity of each image is the simplest way to reduce or suppress activity in the organs surrounding the myocardium [30]. Another method, proposed by Goris et al. as "interpolative background subtraction," is based on the premise that the non-myocardial activity in the cardiac area may be approximated by interpolation of the surrounding activity [31]. This has been criticized by Narahara et al. who removed the heart in dogs and found that the remaining activity was lower than calculated by interpolation [32]. Although this conclusion may also be criticized when extended to a human thorax, it has not been demonstrated that "interpolative background subtraction" provides the true background value. Nevertheless, in our experience, it has proved useful in visualizing ischemia in the inferior ventricular wall, particularly in the anterior projection. Care must be taken, however,

Table 1. Comparison of reliability and performance of analogue and computerized exercise myocardial scintigrams

Images	Detection of coronary artery disease		
	Disagreement (%) between 2 observers (1008 segments)	Sensitivity (%)	Specificity (%)
A. Analogue	17	87	78
B. Systolic computerized	15	96	22
C. Diastolic computerized	17	98	11
D. Total computerized	8	94	78

to exclude abdominal organs of high activity from the background region of interest.

In addition to threshold or interpolative background subtraction, a computer may provide quantitative or semiquantitative analysis of the regional ^{201}Tl myocardial uptake.

We have studied more than 500 patients by ^{201}Tl exercise myocardial scintigraphy using both analogue scintiphotos and images displayed after contrast enhancement obtained by a simple 50% threshold subtraction and delineation of the 75% isocount level. All the regions of the scintigrams below this 75% level were postulated to be hypoactive, and a correlative study with coronary arteriography was used to select the segments of the scintigrams where this hypoactivity actually corresponded to ischemia [33]. The 75% value is similar to the lower normal limits for absolute myocardial uptake quantitation used by Buell et al. [34]. However, it is not applicable in women, since absorption of the 80 keV x-rays by breast tissue may cause hypoactivity in the anterior region of the scintigram.

Computer storage of images combined with ECG synchronization allows construction of ECG-gated myocardial scintigrams [35]. Theoretically, this should improve the resolution by reducing or even suppressing the effects of the cyclic displacement of the heart. This procedure, however, is not often used in stress myocardial scintigraphy because when the counts are collected in only systole or diastole, there is a considerable loss of efficiency. Since all the images must be collected before significant redistribution of ^{201}Tl to the previously ischemic regions, compensation for loss of efficiency by an increase in counting time is not desirable.

In a group of 56 patients, we have compared stress scintigrams simultaneously recorded as: analogue images on Polaroid film; computerized images of systole and diastole obtained by summation of the counts recorded during the second and the fourth quarter of each cardiac cycle, respectively; and total computerized images collected during the whole cardiac cycle. The reliability, the sensitivity and the specificity of these four types of scintigrams are summarized in Table 1. Reliability was evaluated in terms of the percentage disagreement between two independent observers who were asked to classify each of the 18 segments of the 56 patients as normal or hypoperfused, according to our method of segmental analysis described previously [33]. Sensitivity was defined as the percentage of patients with an arteriographically documented coronary stenosis of more than 50% of the arterial diameter in whom an abnormal scintigram was found. Specificity was determined as the percentage of patients without documented stenosis in whom a normal scintigram was found [33].

The percentage disagreement between the two observers was significantly reduced by use of the total computerized images (D) as compared with analogue (A), and gated (B, C) images. The sensitivity of stress myocardial scintigraphy for detection of coronary artery disease was increased by use of both total (D) and gated computerized (B, C) images, but gated images did not provide sufficient specificity because of the nonhomogeneous aspect of scintigrams collected in only one quarter of the heart cycle. Taking the shortest time necessary to collect the scintigrams as a fundamental requirement, it appears that computerized images recorded during the whole cardiac cycle offer the best reliability and performance.

Correlation with Coronary Arteriography

Scintigraphic analysis must proceed with a cautious awareness of possible interpretive errors. First, stress scintigraphy and coronary arteriography do not study precisely the same phenomenon. True stress-induced ischemia may exist in some patients with normal coronary arteries. On the other hand, sufficient blood supply by anterograde or retrograde collateral circulation may prevent myocardial ischemia in the presence of documented coronary stenoses. Moreover, when coronary arteriography is used as the standard for evaluating stress scintigraphy, false-negative or false-positive arteriograms may be interpreted, respectively, as false-positive or false-negative scintigrams. In addition, false-negative stress scintigrams may result from insufficient stress, too long a delay between injection and imaging, or poor image resolution.

Finally, whatever the type of image collected (e.g., analogue, computerized with or without contrast enhancement, threshold or background subtraction) the

Table 2. Sensitivity and specificity of Tl-201 combined rest and stress myocardial scintigraphy for the detection of coronary artery disease

Author	Number of patients	Sensitivity (%)	Specificity (%)	Performance (%)
Bailey [36]	83	75	100	88
Hamilton [37]	137	77	93	85
Meller [38]	55	83	85	84
Ritchie [39]	190	78	88	83
Turner [40]	75[a]	68	97	83
Carillo [41]	55	86	100	93
Verani [42]	82	79	97	88
Lenaers [28]	100[a]	92	86	89

[a] Patients without previous myocardial infarction

Table 3. Detection of coronary artery stenoses by exercise myocardial scintigraphy

	Detection of stenoses on			Detection of CAD
	LAD	LCX	RCA	
A. 150 patients with or without myocardial infarction				
Sensitivity (%)	89	48	78	95
Specificity (%)	83	86	88	83
B. 100 patients without evidence of previous myocardial infarction				
Sensitivity (%)	83	48	63	92
Specificity (%)	88	88	91	86

LAD = left anterior descending artery
LCX = left circumflex artery
RCA = right coronary artery
CAD = coronary artery disease

findings with each technique must be compared with data obtained by invasive methods in order to identify the scintigraphic regions that provide reliable information with each individual technique. For instance, decreased activity in the posterior region on the left lateral view is not reliable when scintigrams are collected with the patient supine [33], but could be indicative of left circumflex or right coronary artery disease when recorded with the patient lying on his right side. In the supine position, the anterior region is near the gamma camera and the posterior region is relatively far away so that it appears hypoactive. When the patient is lying on his right side, both regions are equally far from the gamma camera and no relative hypoactivity is seen in the normal subject. The apical region is often hypoactive even in normal individuals, probably because it is much thinner than other myocardial regions. This hypoactivity on stress myocardial scintigrams must be differentiated from larger defects extending to the anterior, anterolateral, or anteroseptal regions, which are indicative of left anterior descending artery disease [33].

Bearing these reservations in mind, stress myocardial scintigraphy would appear to be a good method for the noninvasive detection of coronary artery disease. Table 2 summarizes the results reported in the literature. Since some investigators used only stress images and others employed both rest and stress scintigrams, all the perfusion defects present after exercise (including defects present at rest) are considered here for purposes of comparison. Sensitivity and specificity are evaluated, as described above, with coronary arteriography used as the reference method. Since there is a balance between the respective values, depending on the threshold chosen to classify the scintigrams as normal or abnormal, their mean value, sometimes referred to as the "performance" of the method, is also listed. Sensitivity ranges from 68 to 92%, specificity from 85 to 100%, and performance from 83 to 93%.

Sensitivity is influenced by the number of significantly narrowed coronary arteries and the presence of previous myocardial damage [36]. Bailey et al. found perfusion defects, present at rest or induced by stress, in 71%, 65%, and 93% of patients with one-vessel, two-vessel, and three-vessel disease, respectively [36]. The distribution of coronary artery lesions also plays an important role. Table 3 shows the sensitivity and specificity of detection of left anterior descending, left circumflex, and right coronary artery disease by exercise myocardial scintigraphy in 150 consecutive patients submitted to coronary arteriography. Stress myocardial scintigraphy is very sensitive to the presence of disease of the left anterior descending artery, less sensitive to disease of the right coronary artery especially when there has been no previous myocardial infarction, and poorly sensitive to disease of the left circumflex artery [28, 33]. The poor sensitivity for detection of left circumflex artery disease has been confirmed by McLaughlin et al. and may be explained by the relatively limited territory supplied by this artery in most patients [29].

Comparison with Exercise ECG

Exercise ECG is designed to provide objective evidence of myocardial stress-induced ischemia by registering specific abnormalities. Most cardiologists agree that an ST-segment horizontal or descending depression of at least 0.1 mV is the best ECG sign of inadequate myocardial blood flow during stress. There is, however, a significant incidence of false-positive and false-negative results, varying widely with the level

Table 4. Comparison between ECG and stress myocardial scintigraphy for the detection of coronary artery disease

Author	Number of patients	Rest or stress defects on scintigrams			Rest Q waves or ischemic stress ST-segment depression		
		Sensitivity (%)	Specificity (%)	Performance (%)	Sensitivity (%)	Specificity (%)	Performance (%)
Bailey [36]	83	75	100	88	65	75	70
Hamilton [37]	137	77	93	85	66	83	75
Turner [40]	75[a]	68	97	83	71	79	75
Verani [42]	82	79	97	88	77	76[b]	77
Lenaers [28]	100[a]	92	86	89	71	71	71

[a] Patients without previous myocardial infarction

[b] Including 38% non-diagnostic exercise ECG (heart rate <85% of maximum)

Table 5. Comparison of Tl-201 exercise myocardial scintigraphy and exercise ECG in 100 patients without previous myocardial infarction

Type of coronary artery disease	Number of patients	Stress ECG		Stress scintigraphy	
		Positive	Negative	Positive	Negative
LAD only	16	7	6	15	1
LCx only	3	2	1	0	3
RCA only	7	5	2	4	3
LAD+LCx	18	14	4	18	0
LCx+RCA	2	2	0	2	0
RCA+LAD	9	6	3	8	1
Three-vessel disease	17	15	2	15	2
None or non-significant (≦50%)	28	8	20	4	24

LAD = left anterior descending artery
LCx = left circumflex artery
RCA = right coronary artery

of stress applied and the prevalence of coronary artery disease in the population studied [43]. Despite the possible variations in exercise ECG results, comparison with exercise scintigraphy is valid when the same exercise test is used for both techniques. Care must be taken, however, to compare either signs of stress-induced ischemia on ECG (ischemic ST-segment depression) and exercise scintigrams (only new defects after exercise, not present at rest) or all signs of myocardial damage, even irreversible ones, thus including Q waves on rest ECG and all defects on exercise scintigrams.

The overall accuracy of stress myocardial scintigraphy in the detection of coronary artery disease is about 10–15% better than the combined rest/stress ECG (Table 4). This performance, however, varies according to the severity and the distribution of the coronary artery disease, as discussed above. We have compared stress ECG and stress scintigraphy in 100 patients without myocardial infarction. The results (Table 5) suggest that stress myocardial scintigraphy is especially more sensitive than stress ECG in detecting disease involving the left anterior descending artery alone or in combination with disease of a second vessel, although the number of patients in each subgroup was not sufficient to draw definite conclusions [28]. An inability to detect disease involving only the left circumflex artery may, however, represent a definite limitation of exercise scintigraphy, since in our series none of three patients was detected.

Finally, although it is always desirable to achieve 90% of predicted maximal heart rate to reduce the incidence of false-negative scintigrams, it appears that even at lower exercise levels, exercise scintigraphy is more sensitive than exercise ECG [36, 42]. Thus, abnormal scintigrams may be recorded even with beta-blocking agents. A normal stress scintigram obtained under these conditions, however, must be considered non-diagnostic and repeated at least 48 hours after last beta-blocking drug administration.

Clinical Applications

Rest/exercise myocardial scintigraphy with ^{201}Tl provides valuable information on regional myocardial perfusion during stress [33]. Therefore, the possible applications are:

1. Noninvasive detection of stress-induced myocardial ischemia related to main coronary artery disease or small vessel disease.
2. Noninvasive prediction of significant disease of the left anterior descending artery in the presence of apparently uncomplicated inferior myocardial infarction.
3. Distinction between true-positive and false-positive electrocardiograms in asymptomatic patients.
4. Evaluation of the myocardial perfusion reserve distal to a documented coronary artery stenosis.
5. Recognition of compromised but viable myocardium before coronary artery bypass surgery.
6. Noninvasive evaluation of myocardial perfusion after coronary artery bypass surgery.

Several authors have recommended the use of ^{201}Tl myocardial scintigraphy during rest and exercise after coronary artery bypass surgery [44–48]. The first reports suggest that it may be a good method for predicting graft closure. Further work will be needed to evaluate its place in long-term follow-up studies of surgically treated and untreated patients.

References

1. Zaret, B.L., Strauss, H.W., Martin, N.D., Wells, S.H., Flamm, M.D.: Noninvasive regional myocardial perfusion with radioactive potassium: Study of patients at rest, with exercise, and during angina pectoris. N. Engl. J. Med. 288:809–812, 1973
2. Zaret, B.L., Stenson, R.E., Martin, N.D., Strauss, H.W., Wells, H.P., McGowan, R.L.: Potassium-43 myocardial perfusion scanning for the noninvasive evaluation of patients with false-positive exercise tests. Circulation 48:1234–1241, 1973
3. Zaret, B.L., Martin, N.D., McGowan, R.L., Strauss, H.W., Wells, H.P., Flamm, M.D.: Rest and exercise potassium-43 myocardial perfusion imaging for the noninvasive evaluation of aortocoronary bypass surgery. Circulation 49:688–695, 1974
4. Martin, N.D., Zaret, B.L., Strauss, H.W., Wells, H.P., Albers, J.: Myocardial imaging using ^{43}K and the gamma camera. Radiology 112:446–448, 1974
5. Berman, D.S., Salel, A.F., DeNardo, G.L., Mason, D.T.: Noninvasive detection of regional myocardial ischemia using rubidium-81 and the scintillation camera: Comparison with stress electrocardiography in patients with arteriographically documented coronary stenosis. Circulation 52:619–626, 1975
6. Botvinick, E.H., Shames, D.M., Gershengorn, K.M., Carlsson, E., Ratshin, R.A., Parmley, W.W.: Myocardial stress perfusion scintigraphy with rubidium-81 versus stress electrocardiography. Am. J. Cardiol. 39:364–371, 1977
7. Lurie, A.J., Salel, A.F., Berman, D.S., DeNardo, G.L., Hurley, E.J., Mason, D.T.: Determination of improved myocardial perfusion after aortocoronary bypass surgery by exercise rubidium-81 scintigraphy. Circulation (Suppl.) 54:III-20–23, 1976
8. Lebowitz, E., Greene, M.W., Bradley-Moore, P., Atkins, H., Ansari, A., Richards, P., Belgrave, E.: ^{201}Tl for medical use. J. Nucl. Med. 14:421–422, 1973
9. Lebowitz, E., Greene, M.W., Fairchild, R., Bradley-Moore, P.R., Atkins, H.L., Ansari, A.N., Richards, P., Belgrave, E.: Thallium-201 for medical use. I. J. Nucl. Med. 16:151–155, 1975
10. Bradley-Moore, P.R., Lebowitz, E., Greene, M.W., Atkins, H.L., Ansari, A.N.: Thallium-201 for medical use. II: Biologic behavior. J. Nucl. Med. 16:156–160, 1975
11. Atkins, H.L., Budinger, T.F., Lebowitz, E., Ansari, A.N., Greene, M.W., Fairchild, R.G., Ellis, K.J.: Thallium-201 for medical use. III: Human distribution and physical imaging properties. J. Nucl. Med. 18:133–140, 1977
12. Nishiyama, H., Sodd, V.J., Adolph, R.J., Saenger, E.L., Lewis, J.T., Gabel, M.: Intercomparison of myocardial imaging agents: ^{201}Tl, ^{129}Cs, ^{43}K, and ^{81}Rb. J. Nucl. Med. 17:880–889, 1976
13. Strauss, H.W., Pitt, B.: Thallium-201 as a myocardial imaging agent. Sem. in Nucl. Med. 7:49–58, 1977
14. Wackers, F.J., Sokole, E.B., Samson, G., van der Schoot, J.B., Lie, K.I., Liem, K.L., Wellens, H.J.: Value and limitations of thallium-201 scintigraphy in the acute phase of myocardial infarction. N. Engl. J. Med. 295:1–5, 1976
15. Gould, K.L., Hamilton, G.W., Lipscomb, K., Ritchie, J.L., Kennedy, J.W.: Method for assessing stress induced regional malperfusion during coronary arteriography: Experimental validation and clinical application. Am. J. Cardiol. 34:557–564, 1974
16. Holman, B.L., Cohn, P.F., See, J.R., Idoine, J., Adams, D.F.: Measurement of regional myocardial blood flow with Xe-133 both at rest and after contrast hyperemia. J. Nucl. Med. 16:536, 1975
17. Weich, H.F., Strauss, H.W., Pitt, B.: The extraction of thallium-201 by the myocardium. Circulation 56:188–191, 1977
18. Love, W.D., Burch, G.E.: Influence of the rate of coronary plasma flow on the extraction of Rb^{86} from coronary blood. Circ. Res. 7:24–30, 1959
19. Holman, B.L.: Radionuclide methods in the evaluation of myocardial ischemia and infarction. Circulation (Suppl.) 53:I-112–119, 1976
20. Strauss, H.W., Harrison, K., Langan, J.K., Lebowitz, E., Pitt, B.: Thallium-201 for myocardial imaging. Relation of thallium-201 to regional myocardial perfusion. Circulation 51:641–645, 1975
21. Pohost, G.M., Zir, L.M., Moore, R.H., McKusick, K.A., Guiney, T.E., Beller, G.A.: Differentiation of transiently ischemic from infarcted myocardium by serial imaging after a single dose of thallium-201. Circulation 55:294–302, 1977
22. Beller, G.A., Pohost, G.M.: Mechanism for thallium-201 redistribution after transient myocardial ischemia (abstract). Circulation (Suppl.) 56:III-141, 1977
23. Burguet, W., Becquevort, P., Dwelshauvers, J., Lenaers, A., Merchie, G.: La scintigraphie du myocarde au ^{201}Tl dans la maladie coronarienne. Radioakt. Isotope Klin. Forsch. 12:457–464, 1976
24. Groch, M.W., Lewis, G.K.: Thallium-201: Scintillation camera imaging considerations. J. Nucl. Med. 17:142–145, 1976
25. Graham, L.S., Poe, N.D., Robinson, G.D.: Collimation for imaging the myocardium. II. J. Nucl. Med. 17:719–723, 1976
26. Cook, D.J., Bailey, I., Strauss, H.W., Rouleau, J., Wagner, H.N., Pitt, B.: Thallium-201 for myocardial imaging: Appearance of the normal heart. J. Nucl. Med. 17:583–589, 1976
27. Council on Rehabilitation, International Society of Cardiology: Exercise test methodology. In: Myocardial Infarction: How to Prevent, How to Rehabilitate, edited by T. Semple. Mannheim, Boehringer, 1973, pp. 55–74

28. Lenaers, A., Becquevort, P., Block, P., van Thiel, E., Ermans, A.M.: Segmental analysis of thallium-201 stress myocardial scintigraphy in patients with and without myocardial infarction. In: World Federation of Nuclear Medicine and Biology, Abstracts, Second International Congress, September 17–21, 1978, Washington, D.C., p. 92
29. McLaughlin, P.R., Martin, R.P., Doherty, P., Daspit, S., Goris, M., Haskell, W., Lewis, S., Kriss, J.P., Harrison, D.C.: Reproducibility of thallium-201 myocardial imaging. Circulation 55:497–503, 1977
30. Strauss, H.W., Pitt, B., Rouleau, J., Bailey, I.K., Wagner, H.N., editors: Physiological and technical factors in myocardial perfusion studies. In: Atlas of Cardiovascular Nuclear Medicine. Saint Louis, The C.V. Mosby Company, 1977, p. 18
31. Goris, M.L., Daspit, S.G., McLaughlin, P., Kriss, J.P.: Interpolative background subtraction. J. Nucl. Med. 17:744–747, 1976
32. Narahara, K.A., Hamilton, G.W., Williams, D.L., Gould, K.L.: Myocardial imaging with thallium-201: An experimental model for analysis of the true myocardial and background image components. J. Nucl. Med. 18:781–786, 1977
33. Lenaers, A., Block, P., van Thiel, E., Lebedelle, M., Becquevort, P., Erbsmann, F., Ermans, A.M.: Segmental analysis of Tl-201 stress myocardial scintigraphy. J. Nucl. Med. 18:509–516, 1977
34. Buell, U., Strauer, B.E., Witte, J.: Segmental analysis of Tl-201 stress myocardial scintigraphy: The problem of using uniform normal values of Tl-201 myocardial uptake. J. Nucl. Med. 18:1240–1241, 1977
35. Planiol, T., Itti, R., Pellois, A., Marchal, C.: Dynamic cardiac scintigraphy with a multi-imaging device. Eur. J. Nucl. Med. 1:187–191, 1976
36. Bailey, I.K., Griffith, L.S., Rouleau, J., Strauss, H.W., Pitt, B.: Thallium-201 myocardial perfusion imaging at rest and during exercise: Comparative sensitivity to electrocardiography in coronary artery disease. Circulation 55:79–87, 1977
37. Hamilton, G., Trobaugh, G., Ritchie, J., Williams, D.: An analysis of the clinical usefulness of thallium-201 for detection of coronary disease based on Bayes theorem (abstract). Circulation (Suppl.) 56:III-140, 1977
38. Meller, J., Rudin, A., Goldsmith, S., Pichard, A.D., Gorlin, R., Teichholz, L.E., Herman, M.V.: Spectrum of exercise 201-thallium myocardial imaging in patients with chest pain and normal coronary angiograms (abstract). Circulation Suppl. 56:III-229, 1977
39. Ritchie, J., Zaret, B., Strauss, W., Pitt, B., Berman, D., Schelbert, H., Ashburn, W., Berger, H., Hamilton, G.: Myocardial imaging with thallium-201 at rest and exercise: A multicenter study (abstract). Circulation Suppl. 56:III-230, 1977
40. Turner, D.A., Battle, W.E., Deshmukh, H., Colandrea, M.A., Snyder, G.J., Fordham, E.W., Messer, J.V.: The predictive value of myocardial perfusion scintigraphy after stress in patients without previous myocardial infarction. J. Nucl. Med. 19:249–255, 1978
41. Carrillo, A.P., Marks, D.S., Pickard, S.D., Khaja, F., Goldstein, S.: Correlation of exercise 201-thallium myocardial scan with coronary arteriograms and the maximal exercise test. Chest 73:321–326, 1978
42. Verani, M.S., Marcus, M.L., Razzak, M.A., Ehrhardt, J.C.: Sensitivity and specificity of thallium-201 perfusion scintigrams under exercise in the diagnosis of coronary artery disease. J. Nucl. Med. 19:773–782, 1978
43. Borer, J.S., Brensike, J.F., Redwood, D.R., Itscoitz, S.B., Passamani, E.R., Stone, N.J., Richardson, J.M., Levy, R.I., Epstein, S.E.: Limitations of the electrocardiographic response to exercise in predicting coronary artery disease. N. Engl. J. Med. 293:367–371, 1975
44. Ritchie, J.L., Narahara, K.A., Trobaugh, G.B., Williams, D.L., Hamilton, G.W.: Thallium-201 myocardial imaging before and after coronary revascularization: Assessment of regional myocardial blood flow and graft patency. Circulation 56:830–836, 1977
45. Verani, M.S., Marcus, M.L., Spoto, G., Rossi, N.P., Ehrhardt, J.C., Razzak, M.A.: Thallium-201 myocardial perfusion scintigrams in the evaluation of aorto-coronary saphenous bypass surgery. J. Nucl. Med. 19:765–772 1978
46. Greenberg, B., Hart, R., Werner, J., Brundage, B., Botvinick, E., Chatterjee, K., Parmley, W.: Thallium-201 stress imaging in the follow-up evaluation of coronary bypass patients (abstract). Circulation (Suppl.) 56:III-230, 1977
47. Narahara, K., Ritchie, J., Williams, D., Hamilton, G.: Pre- and postoperative thallium-201 myocardial imaging: Noninvasive assessment of graft patency and regional myocardial perfusion (abstract). Circulation (Suppl.) 56:III-231, 1977
48. Sbarbaro, J.A., Karunaratne, H., Cantez, S., Harper, P., Resnekov, L.: Tl-201 imaging in the assessment of coronary artery bypass graft (CABG) patency (abstract). Circulation (Suppl.) 56:III-231, 1977

Assessment of Regional Myocardial Blood Flow Using the Inert Gas Washout Technique

P.R. Lichtlen and H.-J. Engel

Division of Cardiology, Department of Internal Medicine, Hannover Medical University, Hannover, FRG

The measurement of myocardial blood flow in man using the inert gas clearance technique is limited to several approaches and is always linked with invasive procedures. As coronary artery disease, the main object of these investigations, has a regional character, the techniques should be able to detect small differences in flow in the individual myocardial areas perfused by the major coronary branches. Sampling of the radiotracer can take place directly from the coronary sinus blood or the great cardiac vein, or indirectly, from the cardiac tissue by placing a gamma scintillation camera over the heart.

At best, coronary sinus sampling will allow only a crude differentiation between flow that originates from the anterior wall and drains into the great cardiac vein, and flow from the posterolateral wall, which drains into the small and middle cardiac vein, into the distal coronary sinus. For this reason, inert gas clearance recorded from the coronary sinus, either after inhalation of argon [5, 63] or helium [35, 36], or after selective intracoronary injection of ^{133}Xe or ^{85}Kr[11], is usually considered to be a global technique, which measures flow from the total left ventricle, including normal and poststenotic areas [36]. In special cases, coronary sinus sampling can result in functional regionalization when helium is used as an indicator [35] and the washout curve is dissected into high and low flow components by compartmental analysis; nevertheless, an exact anatomic correlation is not possible with this method.

Precise localization of areas with different flow levels and, thus, an exact determination of flow to discreet anatomic regions, is possible only with precordial, spatially oriented recording of the isotope activity. Using gamma cameras to map the speed of isotope washout, regionalization of the heart into 400–600 small areas (matrix points) can be achieved, limited only by the resolution of the gamma camera, the size of the heart, and the counting statistics derived from the washout curves.

There are only a few washout techniques that are used in man at the present time:

1. The precordial xenon clearance or residue detection technique, the most widely used technique, and the only one with true clinical applicability [31, 45, 53, 59];

2. The rapid washout technique, using the short-lived isotope krypton-81 [61], which has so far been used mainly for experimental purposes;

3. The tomographic positron camera technique [64], which is still in the early stage of development, but would seem to have great clinical potential.

The following presentation will deal mainly with the precordial xenon clearance technique, its methodology, the criticisms that have been raised about it, and its research as well as clinical applications.

Theoretical and Technical Considerations

Theory of Washout Calculations

Assessment of myocardial blood flow by precordial registration of washout or clearance curves was first performed by Herd [26] in animal studies, and by Ross and co-workers [58, 59], in human subjects. The technique was based on the premise that after an intracoronary bolus injection, the inert gas, dissolved in saline, would rapidly diffuse into the tissue (myocardial, fibrous, and adipose tissue) supplied by the coronary arteries and be washed out from the tissue as a direct function of blood flow. The analysis of the washout function was performed on the basis

Address reprint requests to: Prof. Paul R. Lichtlen, Director, Division of Cardiology, Department of Internal Medicine, Karl-Wiechert Allee 9, D-3000 Hannover, Federal Republic of Germany

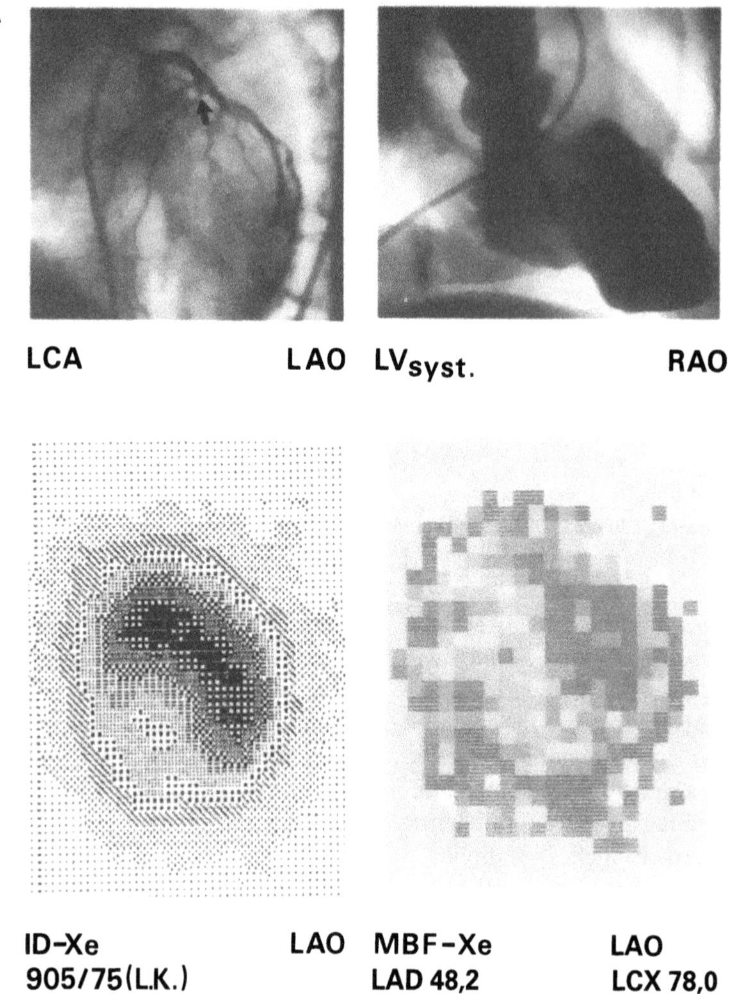

Fig. 1 A. Initial xenon distribution and flow-image after injection of 10 mCi ^{133}Xe into the left coronary artery. *Top left*: Left coronary angiogram in a 40° left anterior oblique projection, which is identical to the flow measurement projection. *Top right*: Left ventricular angiogram in end-systole, 40° right anterior oblique projection. There is greater than 80% obstruction of the left anterior descending artery in its upper third; the left ventricular angiogram shows extensive akinesis involving the anterior wall, the apical area, and the proximal parts of the diaphragmatic wall. *Bottom left*: Initial xenon distribution (40° left anterior oblique projection). Note the high xenon activity in the posterolateral wall, corresponding to the area of perfusion of the left circumflex artery and the almost complete absence in the area perfused by the left anterior descending artery. Black indicates the maximum activity (which is set equal to 100%); the decreasing intensity indicates decreasing activity. *Bottom right:* Color-scan of xenon washout, indicating myocardial blood flow (MBF-Xe) for each matrix point. Red indicates the highest flow values, with flow decreasing in intervals of 10% through orange, yellow, dark-green, light green, and blue. Note the high flow rates in the area perfused by the left circumflex artery (78 ml/min/100 g) and the low values in the region of the left anterior descending artery (48.2 ml/min/100 g). (ID-Xe = initial xenon distribution; LVsyst = end-systolic frame.)

of a monoexponential model applied to the initial slope, following the Kety-Schmidt formula [33] for the exchange of inert gases in the lung and tissue:

$$F/W = \frac{k \times \lambda \cdot 100}{\rho} \text{(ml/min/100 g)}$$

where F/W represents blood flow per 100 g myocardium, λ the blood-myocardium partition coefficient for xenon, indicated by Conn [13] as 0.72 in the normal dog, and ρ the specific gravity of the heart (= 1.05). The rate constant k, the only variable in the equation, is derived from the exponential washout function of any gas [31, 36, 39, 53, 54, 59, 70], and is derived as follows:

$$k = \frac{\ln 2}{T_{1/2}}$$

where $T_{1/2}$ represents the time in minutes required for the count rate to be reduced by 50%. Thus, the only variable to be determined by the scintillation probe or gamma camera is $T_{1/2}$. Throughout the 1960s, this technique was used for recording global myocardial blood flow, with a single scintillation probe located over the heart. The development of gamma scintillation cameras [1], in conjunction with computer image processing made possible a modification of the original technique with registration of multiple time-activity curves attributable to multiple sections of the left ventricular wall, and thus resulted

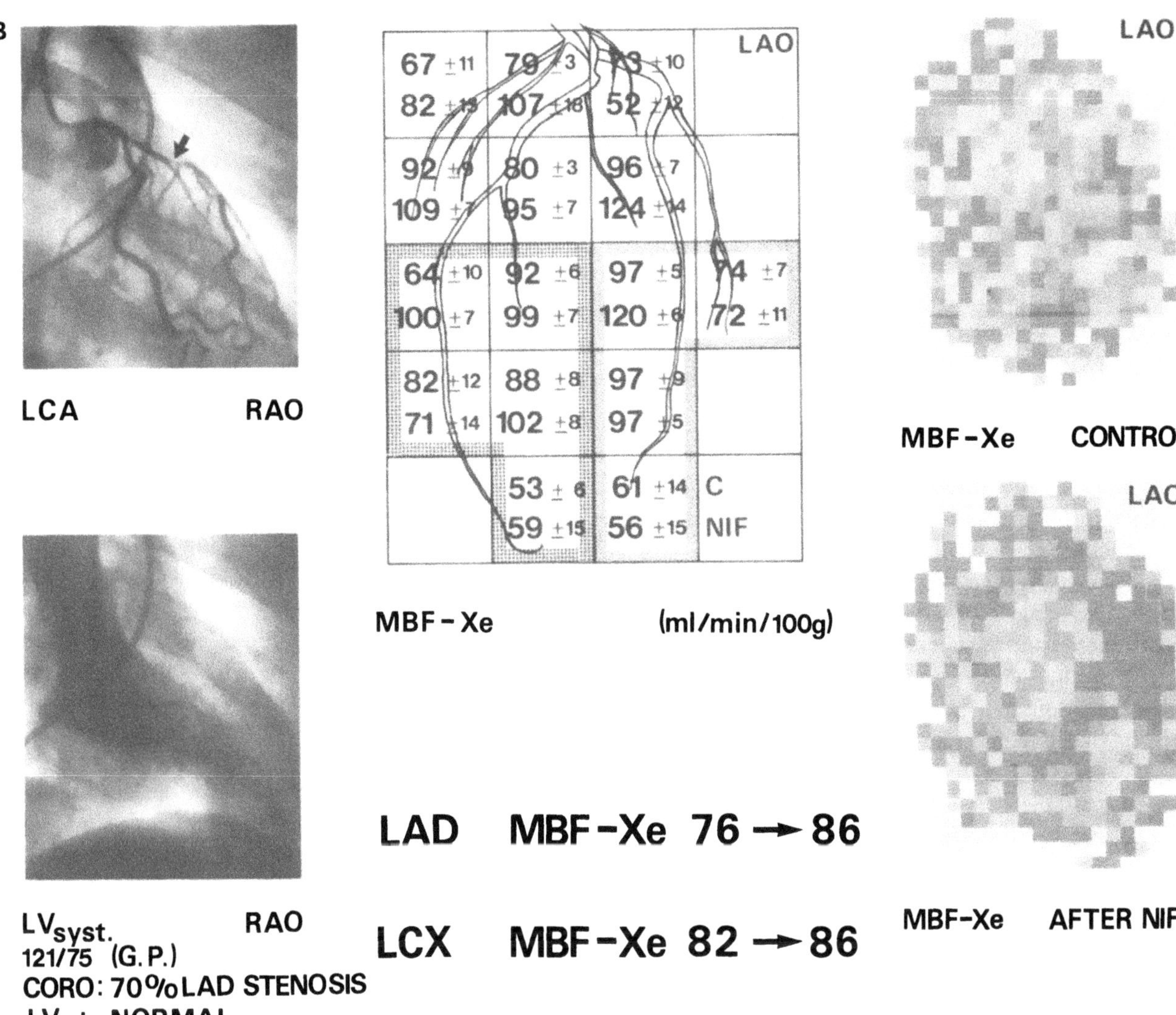

Fig. 1 B. Regional myocardial blood flow recording before and after sublingual administration of 20 mg nifedipine. *Left:* A left coronary and left ventricular angiogram (40° right anterior oblique projection). There is a 70% obstruction of the proximal left anterior descending artery (*arrow*), but left ventricular wall motion is still normal as shown on the end-systolic frame of the left ventricular angiogram (LVsyst). *Middle.* Numerical printout of xenon washout (ml/min/100 g myocardium) for areas of 25 matrix points before (top of each quadrant) and 10 minutes after drug administration (bottom of each quadrant). Flow values are indicated together with their standard deviations. The areas perfused by the left anterior descending (LAD) and left circumflex (LCX) arteries are indicated separately. The flow recording was made in a 40° left anterior oblique projection. *Right.* Color scan before (top) and after nifedipine (bottom). Red indicates the highest, green and blue the lowest flow values. Note that at rest, during control measurements, lower flow values (76 ml/min/100 g) were averaged in the poststenotic area of the left anterior descending artery than in the normal area of the left circumflex artery (86 ml/min/100 g). The color scan also shows the red matrix points as located mainly in the area perfused by the left circumflex artery. After the drug was administered there was a marked increase in flow in both the poststenotic and the normal zone.

in a semi-quantitative estimation of regional myocardial blood flow.

Instrumentation

In our investigations, the xenon gamma-ray emission is detected using a modified gamma camera (Pho/Gamma III, Searle Radiographics, Des Plaines, Ill.) and a low-energy, high-resolution collimator, connected to an external controller (four k memory) and a CDC 1700 computer system (32 k memory, 16 bit word size, two magnetic disc and one tape units). A homogeneous (uniform) field of view is achieved by routine calibration of the equipment.

As a consequence of improved temporal resolution of the gamma camera, the dead time of the whole system is only 4 µsec. The dead time of the system is short enough so that no significant loss of counts occurs at maximal count rates with the doses of the radiotracer used in our studies, eliminating the need for dead-time correction. Data transfer from the camera to the computer is performed in frame mode by a buffered data channel. The time for transfer of each frame is 14 msec.

Procedure of the Hannover Medical School

At Hannover Medical School, the procedure is facilitated by the spatial arrangement of the x-ray unit and the gamma camera, which permits transfer of the patient from the x-ray U-arm to the gamma camera within seconds after intubation of the coronary artery.

The xenon studies are performed in a 40° left anterior oblique projection. This plane permits adequate spatial separation of the distribution of the left anterior descending and the left circumflex arteries, as well as a separation of the free right ventricular wall from the inferior left ventricle in right coronary artery studies. Registration of time-activity curves starts simultaneously with the injection into the left or right coronary artery of 10–20 mCi of ^{133}Xe dissolved in 1 ml of saline. With sequential examinations, background activity, registered during 20 seconds before the injection, is automatically subtracted. The precordial radioactivity is registered for two minutes. The frame length is two seconds during the first minute, and five seconds during the second minute, resulting in a total of 42 frames.

Both the dynamic information derived from the clearance curve and the flow distribution data as displayed by the scintigraphic image of the initial xenon distribution are analyzed. The washout curves are routinely analyzed for each matrix element (0.5×0.5 cm) and for larger areas of 25 matrix points each (2.5×2.5 cm). The rate constant k and the standard deviation of k are calculated by the method of least squares from the initial 30 seconds of the washout curves. For most cases, this approximates the first monoexponential slope of the clearance curve, except with very high flow rates. Rate constants are converted into flow rates (ml/min/100 g) by the Kety-Schmidt equation. The results are displayed numerically for individual matrix elements as well as for the larger areas of 25 matrix points. In addition, a graphic display of the clearance data is obtained as a functional image, indicating the flow values in symbols, that is, in gradations of gray or as different colors [29]. (A typical example is shown in Figure 1).

Information about flow distribution is derived from the scintigraphic image of the precordial activity accumulated during the first ten seconds after xenon injection. Scintigrams of the initial xenon distribution correspond closely to microsphere-perfusion scintigrams [16]; both the xenon distribution image and the microsphere-perfusion image represent static images of flow distribution.

Statistics

The validity of the results requires close attention to statistical considerations. In our procedure, all matrix points that either reach their peak activity later than 15 seconds after injection or attain maximum count rates of less than 15% of the element with maximum activity are rejected from further data processing. For the final analysis, flow rates with standard deviations of 30% or more are disregarded as well. While this method allows the exclusion of extracardiac counts, it may also lead to the loss of areas or matrix points representing very low flow. Under these conditions, the maximum count rate was generally 400–600 counts/matrix element/two sec, with approximately 400–600 matrix elements of the 64×64 matrix qualifying for calculation of cardiac rate constants.

Correlation of Flow and Anatomy

The gamma camera must be integrated into an angiographic x-ray unit in such a manner that its position and that of the image amplifier are exactly parallel. In addition, it is useful to outline the border of the heart by external markers under fluoroscopic control and to perform a coronary angiogram in exactly the same position, usually in a 40° left anterior oblique projection, for correct superimposition of flow image and anatomy [8]. Finally, a scintigram of the xenon activity accumulated over the period from peak activity to 10 seconds later is taken (Fig. 1). This initial distribution image, together with a scintigram following the coronary artery injection of technetium-99m labeled microspheres, usually identifies certain anatomic regions in the functional image, especially the areas perfused by the left anterior descending, left circumflex, or distal right coronary arteries. Fields of uncertain arterial supply or potential overlap of arterial distribution are omitted.

Reproducibility

In ten patients, the xenon injections were repeated after six to eight minutes without any changes in position or interventions altering left ventricular hemodynamics or coronary flow. The regression equation obtained for 118 regions of 25 matrix points ($Y = 3.83 + 0.96\,X$) did not deviate significantly from the line of identity ($r = 0.903$; $p < 0.001$).

Criticisms of the Method

Physical Properties of ^{133}Xe

A major disadvantage in the use of xenon as an indicator for the assessment of myocardial blood flow is its different solubilities in various tissues, especially its high affinity for adipose tissue; this is expressed in the wide range of its partition coefficient, 0.72 for myocardium and 8.0 for fatty tissue [13]. Due to the very low flow through fatty tissue, it is very likely that this affects washout during the first 30 seconds only to a small, statistically negligible degree and primarily affects the later portion of the washout curve. Recirculation and trapping of xenon in the lungs behind the heart are also most likely of minor importance in the early stages of imaging [53, 54, 62].

Diffusibility has also been questioned, especially under high flow conditions [27]. This, however, seems to cause few problems, as animal experiments have shown an excellent correlation between xenon flow and coronary flow, as measured by electromagnetic flowmeters, up to 300 ml/min/100 g myocardium [2, 3]. This is within the limits of flow recorded with precordial xenon clearance, even during heavy exercise [30, 41, 43].

The production of Compton scatter which is responsible for 12.5% of counts registered at a distance of 1.5 cm of water, introduces another source of error [50].

The advantages of using ^{133}Xe are the easy collimation due to low energy gamma emission (81keV) and the low radiation exposure to the patient resulting from the short physical half-life (5.3 days) and the 95% elimination during a single passage through the pulmonary circulation [10, 38, 59]. This also renders handling easy and preferable to, for instance the handling of krypton-85, which has a physical half-life of 11 years.

Theoretical Aspects of Washout Techniques

The theory of flow measurements with any inert gas is based on several assumptions. During the period of recording, arterial inflow and venous outflow must be constant, and the gas in the venous blood and that in the myocardium must be in equilibrium. Furthermore, the gas concentration must be the same throughout its volume of distribution. The requirement of uniform inert gas concentrations in all regions of the heart represents a serious problem, due to the heterogeneity of the coronary flow, especially in coronary disease, where the indicator is predominantly delivered to high flow areas and the saturation period is prolonged in low flow compartments. Global techniques recording a sum of washout curves from individual areas of the heart result in an overestimation of flow, total flow being weighted in favor of areas with high flow. Although this objection concerns mainly global techniques, it also pertains to some extent, to the regional approach. For instance, regional techniques are unable to distinguish between epicardial and endocardial flow because regional washout curves represent global transmural flow to each area. In addition, the spherical geometry of the heart may result in a superimposition of more than one area, e.g., anterior and posterior myocardial segments, especially in the border zone of the heart. This is further accentuated by the attenuation of xenon radiation, resulting in less efficient detection from posterior regions.

Monoexponential analysis of regional washout curves is based on the assumption that flow within the field of view of each matrix element is homogeneous. For various reasons, however, strictly monoexponential washout curves cannot be achieved consistently with presently available technology:

1. The spherical geometry of the heart results in a superimposition of normal and underperfused myocardium within the same field;

2. The transmural heterogeneity of flow [28] cannot be measured;

3. Overlapping between adjacent matrix points results in the smear effect [36]; this cross-over effect increases with increasing distance from the detector; and

4. The inhomogeneity of tissue structures even within small washout zones results in a mixture of various partition coefficients. This is especially true in asynergic areas of the heart where scar tissue is interspersed with residual viable tissue; here, flow will be weighted in favor of the high flow areas and will reflect a falsely high flow value for this zone of old myocardial infarction [53].

By concentrating primarily on the initial slope of the washout curve, the level of error introduced may be kept to a minimum. Thus, monoexponential analysis of the initial washout slope results in a useful estimate of average regional transmural flow, especially when washout is expressed as a rate-constant k or $T_{1/2}$, or demonstrated as a flow image [9, 45, 53, 54]. Moreover, the ability of the capillary circulation to clear a freely diffusible indicator from myocardial tissue is an important observation in its own right, independent of the theories and limitations inherent in the monoexponential analysis and the Kety-Schmidt equation. Important physiologic and pharmacologic conclusions may be derived from a comparison of washout rates of normal versus poststenotic areas in the same patient, or of washout rates before and after pharmacologic or physical interventions in the same patient.

Presently Available Nuclear Medicine Technology

The limitations due to collimation, dead-time, cardiac geometry, and resolution restrict the ability to record precisely the radioactive dynamics in small regions of the heart. Spatial resolution ranges from 8 to 14 mm depending on the distance from the collimator [8, 52]; thus, the areas analyzed must be sufficiently large and at an adequate spatial distance from each other.

Finally, regional flow measurements are valid only if there is a close correlation between the functional blood flow measurements and the anatomic regions of the heart derived from angiography. Evaluation is facilitated when flow of abnormal areas can be compared with flow from normal zones in the same patient.

The practical limitations of the precordial xenon clearance technique include the need for selective intracoronary injection of the tracer and for the coupling of the procedure with coronary angiography, which thus necessitates a well-equipped angiographic and nuclear medicine laboratory. Furthermore, data processing is complex and time-consuming and requires access to sophisticated computer facilities. Nevertheless, much of the knowledge gathered during the last few years on both normal and abnormal coronary blood flow in humans, especially patients with coronary artery disease, is based on this methodology [9, 17, 19, 29, 31, 44–49, 53, 60].

Clinical Results

Normal Flow

In 39 patients with angiographically normal or only mildly diseased coronary arteries (less than 30% obstruction) and normal left ventricular wall motion and hemodynamics, flow to the total left ventricular myocardium averaged 65.9 ml/min/100 g, 64.4 for the area perfused by the left anterior descending artery, and 66.3 ml/min/100 g for the area perfused by the left circumflex artery (Table 1). These values are in excellent agreement with those obtained by other groups using the same technique, who have shown a range of values between 61 and 76 ml/min/100 g (Table 2A [9, 29, 54, 55, 57, 59, 60]). Flow rates recorded over the free wall of the right ventricle (42.7 ml/min/100 g) are significantly lower than those from the left ventricle ($p < 0.0125$) (Table 2B).

Poststeonotic Antegrade Flow

Only in the last few years has it been possible to analyze flow in areas perfused by coronary arteries with critical obstructions and thus characterize the relation between poststenotic flow and left ventricular wall motion in man. The development of gamma cameras with a high spatial resolution was a prerequisite [6].

Figure 2 and Table 3 summarize the observations made in 62 patients with isolated single vessel disease, mostly high-grade (>75%) proximal obstructions of the left anterior descending artery and, in a few cases, of the left circumflex artery.

This group of patients was chosen so that flow to normal and poststenotic segments could be distinguished in the same patient [19, 45]. The data suggest a progressive decrease in poststenotic flow even at rest with increasing severity of luminal obstruction and with increasing impairment of left ventricular wall motion in the same area. Flow at rest depends primarily on wall motion and only secondarily on the severity of obstruction. Flow was not reduced in patients with normal left ventricular wall motion, no matter what the degree of obstruction; normal wall motion in the presence of obstruction greater than or equal to 75% was often associated with collateral vessels. On the other hand, obstructions greater than or equal to 90% were rarely associated with normal wall motion (four of 30 cases only), while half the patients with narrowings between 50 and 75% (nine out of 17 cases) showed normal motion. Thus, obstructions of greater than 90% lead to the development of myocardial infarction with resultant asynergy unless collateralization occurred first.

In the presence of high-grade obstruction, local oxygen demand rather than the obstruction itself controls regional flow. In areas of hypokinetic wall motion, flow is reduced to a significantly greater extent in patients with an electrocardiogram (ECG) diagnostic of myocardial infarction (Q >40 msec or >25% of R-wave) than in those in whom the ECG was normal (Table 4). Obviously, the further reduction in myocardial blood flow in areas with scar tissue is due to the low myocardial oxygen consumption rather than to the degree of obstruction.

The significant reduction in flow in areas with hypokinetic or akinetic wall motion in patients with normal or only mildly (less than 30%) obstructed coronary arteries, but with a typical history and ECG-signs of myocardial infarction also supports this view (Fig. 2). In ten women, most of whom developed a myocardial infarction after taking oral contraceptives, flow in akinetic areas was also reduced by 44%, that is, by the same amount as in patients with myocardial infarction and greater than 75% obstruction in the nutritive artery [17, 19, 47].

These findings are in good agreement with experimental studies, which have shown a decrease in coro-

Table 1. Myocardial blood flow (ml/min/100 g) in patients with normal coronary arteries and normal left ventricular function

Coronary artery	Ventricular area	Myocardial blood flow (ml/min/100 g)	No. of patients
Left coronary artery			
Left anterior descending artery	Anterior wall/interventricular septum	64.4 ± 13.9	39
Left circumflex artery	Lateral wall	66.3 ± 17.3	39
Global left coronary artery	Total left ventricular area	65.9 ± 17.8	39
Right coronary artery			
Right ventricular branches	Free right ventricular wall	42.7 ± 7.1	9
Posterior descending, posterolateral	Diaphragmatic wall of left ventricle	69.1 ± 14.3	7
Global right coronary artery	Total right ventricle + left ventricular LV diaphragmatic segments	52.0 ± 15.6	9

Left coronary artery vs right coronary artery, $p < 0.0125$
Right ventricular branches vs left ventricular, diaphragmatic segment, $p < 0.001$

Table 2A. Resting normal flow values for left ventricular myocardium obtained by the precordial xenon clearance technique

Author	Year	No. of patients	Flow (ml/min/100 g)
Ross [59]	1964	18	61
Pitt [57]	1969	15	76
Lichtlen [40]	1972	21	63.9
Holman [29]	1974	9	73
Mösslacher [55]	1976	10	77.4 for LAD 80.1 for LCx
Cannon [9]	1977	17	64
Maseri [54]	1977	4	63.4[a]
Engel [18]	1977	39	64.4 for LAD 66.3 for LCx 69.1 for distal RCA

[a] $T_{1/2} = 0.75$ minute

LAD = left anterior descending artery
LCx = left circumflex artery
RCA = right coronary artery

Table 2B. Resting normal flow values for right ventricular myocardium obtained by the precordial xenon clearance technique

Author	Year	No. of patients	Flow (ml/min/100 g)
Ross [59]	1964	18	49.7
Pitt [57]	1969	15	48.0
Lichtlen [40]	1972	21	46.2
Engel [18]	1977	48	42.7 for free wall of RV 52.0 for total RCA
Cannon [9]	1977	17	47.0

RV = right ventricle
RCA = right coronary artery

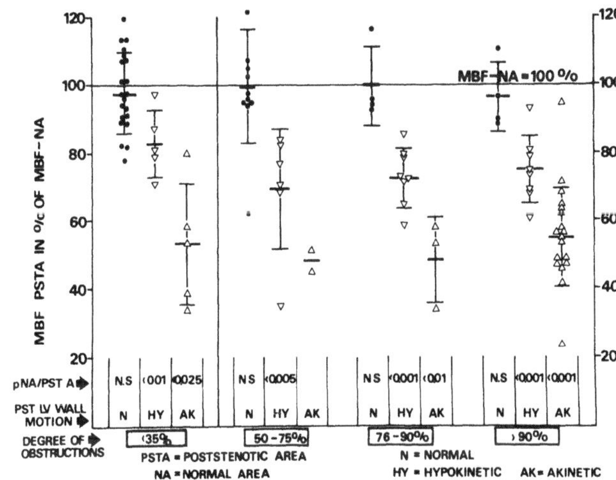

Fig. 2. Relation between poststenotic myocardial blood flow, degree of obstruction, and left ventricular wall motion. Only patients with single-vessel disease were included, allowing a clear comparison between flow in the normal area, set as 100%, and flow in the poststenotic zone indicated as a percentage of the normal area. Coronary obstructions were measured from different projections by a vernier with an accuracy of 0.05 mm, the tip of the catheter being the reference. (MBF-NA = flow in the normal area [= 100%], MBF-PSTA = flow in the poststenotic area). Left ventricular wall motion was assessed from the percentage systolic shortening of six hemiaxes, shortenings greater than 25% being considered as normal, between 25 and 10% as hypokinetic, and below 10% as akinetic. (Black circles = flow in poststenotic areas with normal wall motion; reversed triangles = flow in hypokinetic zones, upright triangles = flow in akinetic zones.)

nary flow when luminal narrowing reaches 75–80% [25, 56, 69]. The few other studies that have measured poststenotic flow in man with other techniques have also defined critical obstruction at rest as a 70–80% narrowing [7, 9, 54].

Table 3. Effect or coronary obstruction and segmental wall motion on regional myocardial blood flow with flow rates in the poststenotic (asynergic) left ventricular wall regions expressed as a percentage of flow in the respective normal regions where flow was set as 100%

Left ventricular poststenotic wall motion	Degree of coronary artery obstruction				Average values
	<35%	50–75%	76–90%	>90%	
Normal[a]	100%	99.9±16.7% (10) n.s.[f]	100.0±11 3% (4) n.s.	96.5±10.2% (4) n.s.	99.2±13.8% (18) n.s.
Hypokinetic[b]	83.2± 9.8% (5)[d] $p<0.01$[e]	69.5±17.9% (6) $p<0.005$	72.5± 8.8% (7) $p<0.0005$	75.3± 9.7% (8) $p<0$ 0005	74.8±12.1% (26) $p<0.0005$
Akinetic[c]	53.5±18.4% (5) $p<0.0025$	48.3± 4.8% (2) $p<0.025$	48.5±12.5% (3) $p<0.01$	55.5±14.7% (18) $p<0.0005$	54.6±15.1% (18) $p<0.0005$
		84.0±24.8% (18) $p<0.01$	75.2±21.1% (14) $p<0.0005$	66.5±19.4% (30) $p<0.0005$	

[a] Systolic shortening of 6 hemiaxes >25%
[b] Systolic shortening of 6 hemiaxes 25–10%
[c] Systolic shortening of 6 hemiaxes <10%
[d] Numbers in parentheses indicate numbers of patients
[e] Results of paired t-test
[f] n.s.= not significant

Table 4. Percentage decrease in regional myocardial blood flow in asynergic areas of the left ventricle with and without ECG signs of old myocardial infarction

ECG diagnosis	Left ventricular asynergic areas				
	Hypokinetic[a]			Akinetic[b]	
	No. of patients	Decrease in regional blood flow	Average systolic shortening	No. of patients	Decrease in regional blood flow
Myocardial infarction	7	31.9%	12.9%	25	47.1%
Normal	11	19.9%[c]	18.4%	3[c]	40.2%

[a] Systolic shortening of 6 hemiaxes of 10–25% (normal >25%)
[b] Systolic shortening of 6 hemiaxes of less than 10%
[c] $P<0.05$; difference MI vs normal

Poststenotic Collateral Flow

Collateral flow seems to behave like antegrade flow at rest, with its rate highly dependent on segmental wall motion [66]. In our experience with 37 patients with collaterals (in 28 instances, to the left anterior descending artery) flow averaged 57 ml/min/100 g myocardium and thus was only slightly lower than normal. In eight areas with normal wall motion, collateral flow averaged 69.3 ml/min/100 g at rest, while in hypokinetic ($n=11$) and akinetic areas ($n=18$), collateral flow was significantly lower, i.e., 60.6 and 53.1 ml/min/100 g, respectively ($p<0.0025$). When tested with dipyridamole (0.5 mg/kg intravenously), a 50% increase was observed (Fig. 3 [42]), indicating that at rest, coronary reserve was not exhausted, a phenomenon also described by Maddox et al. [51] during contrast hyperemia.

Bypass Flow

The precordial xenon clearance technique, with injection directly into the grafts, is ideally suited to record bypass flow. In a study of 26 patients [39], normal resting values of graft flow were demonstrated to average 58 ml/min/100 g for left anterior descending artery grafts, and 47 ml/min/100 g for right coronary artery grafts. In ten patients, flow during moderate exercise (average oxygen consumption 1250 ml/min,

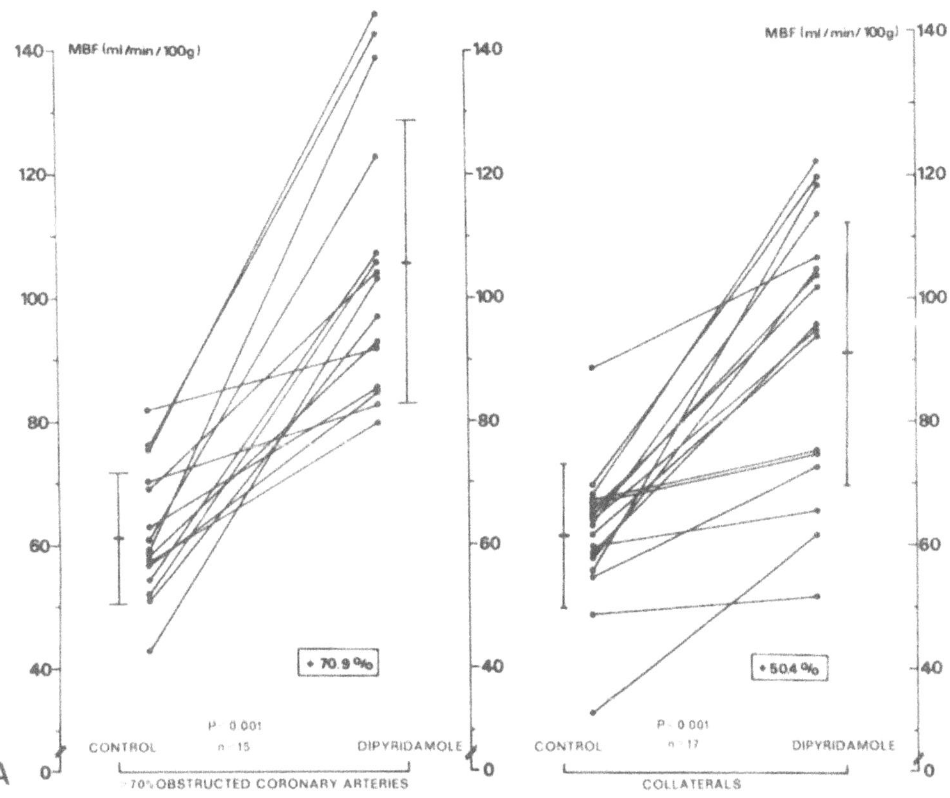

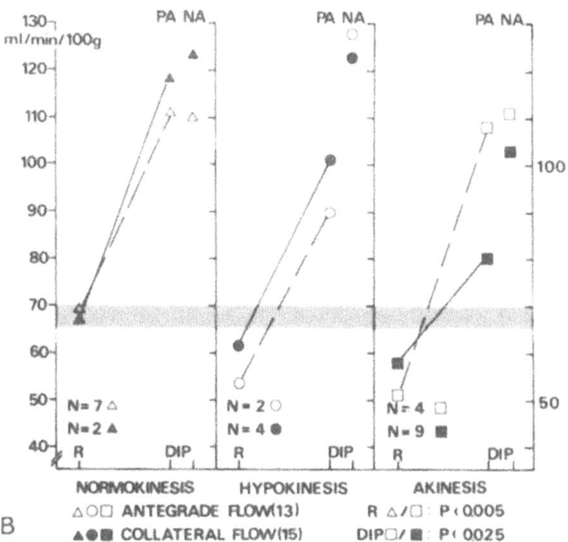

Fig. 3A and B. A Antegrade and retrograde poststenotic, (collateral) blood flow before and after the intravenous injection of 0.5 mg/kg dipyridamole. *Left.* Antegrade flow in areas perfused by coronary arteries with greater than 70% obstructions. Dipyridamole led to a 71% flow increase. *Right:* Flow in coronary arteries perfused entirely by collaterals, mainly the left anterior descending artery. Note that at rest poststenotic flow was identical in arteries perfused antegrade or by collaterals and that after dipyridamole, although the flow increase was slightly higher in the former group, the difference between antegrade and collateral flow was not significant. However, the maximal values achieved were still approximately 50% lower than those observed in patients with normal coronary arteries and left ventricular function, where flow under dipyridamole usually reaches values of 200 ml/min/100 g or more. **B** Regional myocardial blood flow before and after dipyridamole in poststenotic and normal areas in relation to the type of perfusion and left ventricular wall motion. Antegrade and collateral flow were identical except in akinetic zones. There was a progressive decrease in resting flow and in flow after dipyridamole between patients with normokinetic left ventricular wall motion and those with hyperkinetic and akinetic zones. Furthermore, in the latter, flow in normal regions was higher than in poststenotic zones. (Hatched area = normal resting flow; PA = poststenotic area, NA = normal area.)

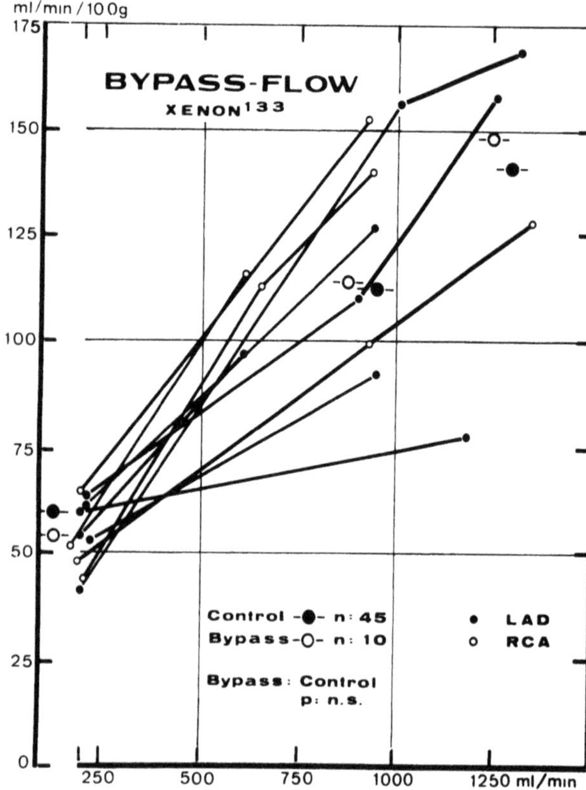

Fig. 4. Global myocardial blood flow at rest and during exercise in areas perfused by coronary artery bypass grafts and normal coronary arteries. For this determination, xenon was injected directly into the graft. Note that graft flow during exercise was equal to flow in areas perfused by normal coronary arteries (obstruction less than 30%) for this work load.

corresponding to approximately 70 W) increased to more than 140 ml/min/100 g (Fig. 4), a rise in flow equal to that found in the normal population [30, 43].

Flow after Drug Interventions

The investigation of the regional inert gas clearance after various antianginal drugs has led to a better understanding of their effect on coronary flow in poststenotic, potentially ischemic areas in patients with coronary artery disease (Table 5). Although, for technical reasons, these studies were performed at rest, in the absence of angina, they help clarify the mechanism of most of the typical antianginal drugs such as nitrates, betablockers, and calcium antagonists.

Nitrates

A highly significant decrease in flow ($p<0.005$) was observed in our group of 25 patients with coronary artery disease, both in the poststenotic (−14%) and in the normal areas (−7%) after the sublingual administration of 0.8 mg nitroglycerin. This decrease in poststenotic resting flow, which has also been shown by other investigators [12] was, in our experience, independent of the degree of obstruction or improvement of wall motion [44]. This is in contrast to findings by Dirschinger [14], who described an increase or no change in poststenotic flow in zones with improved contraction.

The following observations support our view that a reduction in myocardial oxygen consumption rather than an increase in regional myocardial blood flow is the primary antianginal mechanism of nitroglycerin: In ten patients studied during pacing-induced angina [20], flow was reduced in both normal and poststenotic areas after nitroglycerin, while the patients experienced relief of angina pectoris and ST-segment depression was decreased. Since flow reduction in normal areas was more pronounced than in poststenotic zones, the pattern of regional myocardial blood flow was more homogeneous following nitroglycerin administration, a phenomenon also observed with thallium-201 myocardial scintigraphy during exercise [67].

Betablockers

After betablockade, resting coronary flow in both poststenotic and normal areas also shows a significant decrease (−17% and −13%, respectively, $p<0.001$), which is again independent of both the severity of obstruction and the status of wall motion [15, 21, 44, 48, 68]. This change, however, is not associated with an improvement of regional wall motion. These results confirm the traditional concept that the beneficial action of betablockade is based on a decrease in local oxygen demand rather than an increase in blood supply [4, 65]. After both nitrates and betablockers, an intramural redistribution of flow at the expense of the subepicardial myocardium was described in animal experiments [4, 65]; this effect cannot be detected by the xenon inert gas clearance technique, which only measures transmural flow.

Calcium Antagonists

Calcium antagonists, such as nifedipine and verapamil, have been recently introduced for antianginal treatment. Recordings of regional myocardial blood flow after nifedipine [45] showed a mild, significant increase 15 minutes after sublingual administration of 20 mg (Fig. 1 B), which averaged 18% in the poststenotic and 11% in the normal zones and was again

Table 5. Myocardial blood flow, coronary resistance, aortic pressure, heart rate, and pressure rate product in patients with coronary artery disease (CAD pts) and normal subjects (controls) after administration of various drugs

		Myocardial blood flow (ml/min/100 g)			Aortic pressure[a] (mm Hg)			Heart rate b/min	Pressure rate product[a] (mm Hg/min)	Total coronary resistance of normal areas (mm Hg/ ml/min/100 g)
		CAD patients		Controls	Systolic	Diastolic	Mean			
		Post-stenotic areas	Normal areas							
Nitroglycerin		$N=25$	$N=21$	$N=12$						
(22 CAD pts,	before	60.6±15.7	71.8±17.8	67.8±17.2	125	74	96	71	89.297±21.164	1.385±0.335
12 controls)	after	52.3±13.7	66.9±19.0	59.5±19.1	111	70	86	79	88.183±20.313	1.355±0.362
	change	−13.8%	−6.8%	−12.3%	−11.2%	−5.4%	−10.4%	+11.3%	−1.3%	−2.2%
	$p<$	0.005	0.0025	0.0025			0.001	0.001	n.s[b]	n.s
Atenolol		$N=17$	$N=17$	$N=9$						
(17 CAD pts,	before	58.0±12.3	67.7±9.8	64.8±19.1	129	78	98	72	92.870±19.932	1.521±0.227
9 controls)	after	48.3±13.3	58.9±11.5	55.2±15.7	124	75	95	64	80.048±18.636	1.705±0.284
	change	−16.7%	−13.0%	−14.8%	−3.9%	−3.9%	−3.1%	−11.1%	−13.8%	+12.1%
	$p<$	0.001	0.001	0.025			0.001	0.0005	0.001	
Dipyridamole		$N=15$	$N=9$	$N=2$						
(10 CAD pts,	before	59.8±14.8	59.7±13.1	49.2	132	76	97	76	98.529±19.821	1.642±0.435
2 controls)	after	91.5±21.0	103.2±24.5	148.0	120	70	89	88	104.835±23.514	0.792±0.237
	change	+52.9%	+72.9%	+200%	−9.1%	−7.9%	−8.3%	+15.8%	+6.4%	−51.8%
	$p<$	0.001	0.001				0.001	0.001	0.05	0.001
Nifedipine		$N=10$	$N=10$	$N=7$						
(10 CAD pts,	before	58.8±13.0	70.8±19.9	67.7±19.4	131	73	96	79	104.027±24.495	1.541±0.544
7 controls)	after	69.6±15.6	78.7±14.4	81.3±18.7	114	67	87	88	100.253±23.273	1.113±0.313
	change	+18.4%	+11.2%	+20.0%	−13%	−8.2%	−9.4%	+11.1%	−3.4%	−27.8%
	$p<$	0.05	0.05	0.05			0.001	0.001	n.s	n.s

[a] Includes CAD patients and normal subjects
[b] Not significant

independent of the degree of obstruction or wall motion impairment ($p<0.05$). This rise in flow is of relatively short duration, lasting up to 30 minutes after sublingual and only up to three minutes after the intracoronary administration of 0.1mg nifedipine, which leads to an increase in flow of 100%.

These observations concerning flow changes after various drugs, although recorded at rest, lead to several conclusions:

1. An antianginal effect can be achieved both with drugs that either mildly lower or increase poststenotic flow, which suggests that the effect of these drugs on the coronary system is not their primary antianginal mechanism, although it may provide some effect.

2. Antianginal drugs that are truly effective do not abolish coronary reserve; coronary resistance is unchanged after nitrates, increased after betablockade, and only midly decreased after calcium antagonists. In situations of increased oxygen demand, such as exercise [41], the drugs do not inhibit a further rise in flow, yet allow additional coronary arteriolar dilatation. In contrast, the potent coronary vasodilator dipyridamole increases poststenotic transmural flow maximally at rest (Table 5), thus abolishing autoregulation and producing angina pectoris in patients with coronary artery disease [46].

Conclusions

The precordial xenon clearance technique produces a dynamic image of coronary blood flow and provides a precise determination of flow per unit mass, expressed as either $T_{1/2}$, the rate constant k, or in ml/min/100 g myocardium. The methodologic and technical problems of the technique represent serious limitations to its clinical application to the study of regional as well as global flow. Nevertheless, a number of studies have described regional flow in patients with coronary artery disease at rest and during pacing-induced tachycardia and angina [9, 54], regional flow following administration of various drugs [29, 44] collateral flow [22, 45, 66], and flow in bypass grafts [23, 37, 39]. These studies have shown an approximate quantitation of regional flow in coronary patients, especially in the presence of well-defined underperfused and normal, control areas in the same patient; thus, this technique is most informative in cases of single-vessel disease.

Due to the extensive technical apparatus involved and the related costs, the xenon residue detection technique remains an investigative procedure and cannot be recommended for routine clinical use. Nevertheless, it represents an important tool in the determination of regional, functional flow in patients with coronary heart disease. When combined with coronary arteriography and studies increasing myocardial oxygen consumption to the point of ischemia, such as rapid atrial pacing, it may also be used to define patients who are suitable candidates for bypass surgery.

Acknowledgment. The authors like to express their thanks to Prof. Hundeshagen and his coworkers from the Department of Nuclear Medicine for the continuing support in these studies.

References

1. Anger, H.O.: Gamma-ray and positron scintillation camera. Nucleonics 21:56–68, 1963
2. Bassingthwaighte, J.B., Strandell, T., Donald, D.E.: Estimation of coronary blood flow by washout of diffusible indicators. Circ. Res. 23:259–278, 1968
3. Bassingthwaighte, J.B.: Physiology and theory of tracer washout techniques for the estimation of myocardial blood flow: Flow estimation from tracer washout. Progr. Cardiovasc. Dis. 20:165–189, 1977
4. Becker, L., Pitt, B.: Regional myocardial blood flow, ischemia and antianginal drugs. Ann. Clin. Res. 3:353–361, 1971
5. Bretschneider, H.J., Cott, L., Hilgert, G., Probst, R., Rau, G.: Gaschromatographische Trennung und Analyse von Argon als Basis einer neuen Fremdgasmethode zur Durchblutungsmessung von Organen (abstract). Verh. dtsch. Ges. Kreislaufforschg. 32:267, 1966
6. Budinger, T.F., Rollo, F.D.: Physics and instrumentation. Progr. Cardiovasc. Dis. 20:19–53, 1977
7. Bunnell, T.L., Klocke, F.J., Greene, D.G., Arani, D., Tandon, R., Oliveros, R., Wittenberg, S.M.: Effects of isolated left anterior descending coronary artery stenosis on coronary blood flow (abstract). J. Clin. Invest. 53:13a, 1974
8. Cannon, P.J., Haft, J.I., Johnson, P.M.: Visual assessment of regional myocardial perfusion utilizing radioactive xenon and scintillation photography. Circulation 40:277–288, 1969
9. Cannon, P.J., Weiss, M.B., Sciacca, R.R.: Myocardial blood flow in coronary artery disease: Studies at rest and during stress with inert gas washout techniques. Progr. Cardiovasc. Dis: 20:95–120, 1977
10. Chidsey, C.A., Fritts, H.H., Hardewig, A.: Fate of radioactive krypton (Kr^{85}) introduced intravenously in man. J. Appl. Physiol. 14:63–68, 1959
11. Cohen, L.S., Elliott, W.C., Gorlin, R.: Measurement of myocardial blood flow using krypton-85. Am. J. Physiol. 206:997–999, 1964
12. Cohn, P.F., Maddox, D., Holman, B.L., Markis, J.E., Adams, D.F., See, J.R., Idoine, J.: Effects of subliqually administered nitroglycerin on myocardial blood flow in patients with coronary artery disease. Am. J. Cardiol. 39:672–678, 1977
13. Conn, H.L.: Equilibrium distribution of radioxenon in tissue: Xenon-hemoglobin association curve. J. Appl. Physiol. 16:1065–1070, 1961
14. Dirschinger, J., Fleck, E., Redl, A., Brandt, R., Späth, M., Mannes, G., Recke, S., Hall, D., Rudolph, W.: Effects of sodium nitroprusside and isosorbiddinitrate on regional myocardial blood flow in patients with coronary artery disease and left ventricular asynergy. Herz 2:71–74, 1977
15. Dirschinger, J., Fleck, E., Rudolph, W.: Die Bedeutung der Herzfrequenzsenkung für die Wirkung von Betarezeptorenblockern bei koronarer Herzerkrankung (abstract). Z. Kardiol. 67:227, 1978
16. Engel, H.J., Heim, R., Liese, W., Hundeshagen, H., Lichtlen, P.: Regional myocardial perfusion at rest in coronary disease assessed by microsphere scintigraphy and inert gas clearance (abstract). Am. J. Cardiol. 37:134, 1976
17. Engel, H.J., Hundeshagen, H., Lichtlen, P.: Transmural myocardial infarction in young women taking oral contraceptives. Evidence of reduced regional coronary flow in spite of normal coronary arteries. Br. Heart J. 39:477–484, 1977
18. Engel, H.J.: Regionale Myokarddurchblutung. Habilitation, Hannover 1977 (unpublished data)
19. Engel, H.J., Lichtlen, P.R., Hundeshagen, H.: Effects of coronary obstructions and segmental LV dysfunction on regional myocardial blood flow (abstract). Circulation 55/56:(Suppl. III) 10, 1977
20. Engel, H.J., Wolf, R., Hundeshagen, H., Lichtlen, P.: Einfluss von Nitroglyzerin auf die regionale Myokarddurchblutung bei Patienten mit pacing-induzierter Myokardischämie (abstract). Z. Kardiol. 68:283, 1979
21. Fleck, E., Dirschinger, J., Redl, A., Loracher, C., Hall, D., Froer, K.L., Rudolph, W.: Alterations in regional myocardial blood flow and ventricular function induced by betablocking agents and calcium antagonists in patients with coronary artery disease. Herz 2:75–80, 1977
22. Frick, M.H., Valle, M., Korhola, O.: Analysis of coronary collaterals in ischemic heart disease by angiography during pacing-induced ischemia. Br. Heart J. 38:186, 1976
23. Goldberg, A.D., Crawley, J.C.W., Raftery, E.B., Yacoub, M.H.: Myocardial blood flow following saphenous vein bypass surgery. Circulation 51/52:(suppl. I) 215–219, 1975
24. Gould, K.L., Lipscomb, K., Hamilton, G.W.: Physiologic basis for assessing critical coronary stenosis. Instantaneous flow response and regional distribution during coronary hyperemia as measures of coronary flow reserve. Am. J. Cardiol. 33:87–94, 1974
25. Gould, K.L., Lipscomb, K.: Effects of coronary stenoses on coronary flow reserve and resistance. Am. J. Cardiol. 34:48–55, 1974
26. Herd, J.A., Hollenberg, M., Thorburn, G.D., Kopald, H.H., Barcher, A.C.: Myocardial blood flow determined with krypton^{85} in unanesthetized dogs. Am. J. Physiol. 203:122–124, 1962
27. Hirzel, H.O., Krayenbühl, H.P.: Validity of the ^{133}Xenon method for measuring coronary blood flow: Comparison with coronary sinus outflow determined by an electromagnetic flowprobe. Pflueger's Arch. 349:159–169, 1974
28. Hoffman, J.I.E., Buckberg, G.D.: Transmural variations in myocardial perfusion. In: Progress in Cardiology, edited by P.N. Yu and J.F. Goodwin, Philadelphia, Lea & Febiger, 1976, pp. 37–89
29. Holman, B.L., Adams, D.F., Jewitt, D., Eldh, P., Idoine, J., Cohn, P.F., Gorlin, R., Adelstein, S.J.: Measuring regional myocardial blood flow with ^{133}Xe and the Anger camera. Radiology 112:99–107, 1974
30. Holmberg, S., Serzysko, W., Varnauskas, E.: Coronary circulation during heavy exercise in control subjects and patients with

coronary heart disease. Acta Med. Scand. 190:465–480, 1971

31. Hundeshagen, H., Geisler, S., Dittmann, P., Lichtlen, P., Engel, H.J.: Quantitative scintigraphic display of myocardial blood flow: Technique and clinical evaluation. Eur. J. Nucl. Med. 1:107–115, 1976
32. Kety, S.S., Schmidt, C.F.: The determination of cerebral blood flow in man by the use of nitrous oxide in low concentrations. Am. J. Physiol. 143:53–66, 1945
33. Kety, S.S.: Theory and applications of exchange of inert gas at lungs and tissues. Pharmacol. Rev. 3:1–41, 1951
34. Klocke, F.J., Rosing, D.R., Pittman D.E.: Inert gas measurements of coronary blood flow. Am. J. Cardiol. 23:548–555, 1969
35. Klocke, F.J., Bunnell, I.L., Greene, D.G., Wittenberg, S.M., Visco, J.P.: Average coronary blood flow per unit weight of left ventricle in patients with and without coronary artery disease. Circulation 50:547–559, 1974
36. Klocke, F.J.: Clinical measurements of coronary blood flow. In: Progress in Cardiology, edited by P.N. Yu and J.F. Goodwin. Philadelphia, Lea & Febiger, 1976, pp. 91–140
37. Korbuly, D.E., Formanek, A., Gypser, G., Moore, R., Ovitt, T.W., Tuna, N., Amplatz, K.: Regional myocardial blood flow measurements before and after coronary bypass surgery. Circulation 52:38–45, 1975
38. Lassen, N.A.: Assessment of tissue radiation dose in clinical use of radioactive inert gases with examples of absorbed doses from 3-H, 83-Kr, 133-Xe. Minerva Nucl. 8:211–217, 1964
39. Lichtlen, P., Moccetti, T., Halter, J., Schönbeck, M., Senning, A.: Postoperative evaluation of myocardial blood flow in aorta-to-coronary artery vein bypass grafts using the xenon-residue detection technic. Circulation 46:445–455, 1972
40. Lichtlen, P., Moccetti, T., Halter, J.: Myocardial blood flow in man as shown by the precordial xenon-clearance technique. In: Myocardial Blood Flow in Man: Methods and Significance in Coronary Disease, edited by A. Maseri. Torino, Minerva Medica, 1972, pp. 309–320
41. Lichtlen, P., Halter, J., Gattiker, K.: The effect of Isosorbiddinatrate on coronary flow, coronary resistance and left ventricular dynamics under exercise in patients with coronary artery disease. Basic Res. Cardiol. 69:402–421, 1974
42. Lichtlen, P.: Coronary and left ventricular dynamics under nifedipine in comparison to nitrates, betablocking agents and dipyridamole. In: Second International Adalat Symposium: New Therapy of Ischemic Heart Disease, edited by W. Lochner, W. Braasch, and G. Kroneberg. Berlin, Heidelberg, New York, Springer, 1975, pp. 212–224
43. Lichtlen, P.R.: Myocardial blood flow during exercise in patients with coronary artery disease. Herz 2:31–37, 1977
44. Lichtlen, P., Engel, H.J., Hundeshagen, H.: Regional myocardial blood flow in normal and poststenotic areas after nitroglycerin, betablockade (atenolol), coronary dilatation (dipyridamole) and calcium antagonism (nifedipine). Herz 2:81–86, 1977
45. Lichtlen, P.R., Engel, H.J., Hundeshagen, H.: Clinical application and results of the assessment of coronary blood flow by the regional precordial xenon residue detection technique. Nucl. Med. 17:161–171, 1978
46. Lichtlen, P.R., Wolf, R., Engel, H.J., Hundeshagen, H.: Coronary dilatory reserve of severely obstructed coronary arteries and collaterals (abstract). Circulation 57/58:(Suppl. II) 193, 1978
47. Lichtlen, P.R., Engel, H.J.: Angiographic aspects of coronary heart disease in young women. In: Coronary Heart Disease in Young Women, edited by M.F. Oliver, Edinburgh, Churchill Livingstone, 1978, pp. 80–85
48. Lichtlen, P.R., Engel, H.J., Amende, I., Hundeshagen, H.: Effect of betablockade on regional myocardial blood flow in coronary heart disease. International Symposium on Betablockade, Manila, 1978 (in press)
49. Lichtlen, P.R., Engel, H.J., Wolf, R., Amende, I.: The effect of the calcium antagonistic drug nifedipine on coronary and left ventricular dynamics in patients with coronary heart disease. Symposium on the Effect of Calcium-Antagonists, Frankfurt, 1978 (in press)
50. McIntyre, W.J., Cannon, P.J., Ashburn, W.L.: Measurements of regional myocardial perfusion. In: Quantitative Nuclear Cardiology, edited by R.H. Pierson, J.P. Kriss and R.H. Jones. New York, John Wiley and Sons, 1975, p. 170
51. Maddox, D.E., See, J.R., Holman, B.L., Adams, D.F., Cohn, P.F.: Effect of coronary collaterals on regional myocardial blood flow (abstract). Circulation 53/54:(Suppl. II) 231, 1976
52. Maseri, A., Mancini, P., L'Abbate, A.: Method for regional dynamic study of myocardial blood flow in man. J. Nucl. Biol. Med. 15:54–57, 1971
53. Maseri, A.: Radioactive tracer techniques for evaluating coronary flow. In: Progress in Cardiology, edited by P.N. Yu and J.F. Goodwin, Philadelphia, Lea & Febiger, 1976, pp. 141–168
54. Maseri, A., L'Abbate, A., Pesola, A., Michelassi, C., Marzilli, M., De Nes, M.: Regional myocardial perfusion in patients with atherosclerotic coronary artery disease, at rest and during angina pectoris induced by tachycardia. Circulation 55:423–433, 1977
55. Mösslacher, H., Slany, J., Imhof, H.: Correlation between coronary angiography and determination of regional myocardial perfusion in coronary patients using the xenon clearance. In: Coronary Angiography and Angina Pectoris, edited by P.R. Lichtlen. Stuttgart, Thieme, 1976, pp. 284–291
56. Nakamura, M., Matsuguchi, H., Mitsutake, A., Kikuchi, Y., Takeshita, A., Nakagaki, O., Kuroiwa, A.: The effect of graded coronary stenosis on myocardial blood flow and left ventricular wall motion. Basic Res. Cardiol. 72:479–491, 1977
57. Pitt, A., Friesinger, G.C., Ross, R.S.: Measurement of blood flow in the right and left coronary artery bed in humans and dogs using the ^{133}Xenon technique. Cardiovasc. Res. 3:100–106, 1969
58. Ross, R.S., Lichtlen, P.R., Bernstein, L., Ginn, W.M., Ueda, K.: Selective coronary arteriography in man, correlated with clinical electrocardiographic and physiological studies (abstract). Circulation 28:793, 1963
54. Ross, R.S., Ueda, K., Lichtlen, P.R., Rees, J.R.: Measurement of myocardial blood flow in animals and man by selective injection of radioactive inert gas into the coronary arteries. Circ. Res. 15:28–41, 1964
60. Rudolph, W., Fleck, E., Dirschinger, J., Redl, A.: Regional myocardial blood flow determined by the ^{133}Xenon washout technique with respect to coronary artery stenoses and wall motion abnormalities. Herz 2:16–22, 1977
61. Selwyn, A., Fox, K., Forse, G., Steiner, R.: Disturbances of regional myocardial perfusion in patients with coronary artery disease (abstract). Am. J. Cardiol. 43:432, 1979
62. Shaw, D.J., Pitt, A., Friesinger, G.C.: Autoradiographic study of the ^{133}Xenon disappearance method for measurement of myocardial blood flow. Cardiovasc. Res. 6:286–276, 1971
63. Tauchert, M., Kochsiek, K., Heiss, H.W., Strauer, B.E., Kettler, D., Reploh, H.D., Rau, G., Bretschneider, H.J.: Measurement of coronary blood flow in man by the Argon method. In: Myocardial Blood Flow in Man: Methods and Significance in Coronary Disease, edited by A. Maseri. Torino, Minerva Medica, 1972, pp. 139–144
64. Weiss, E.S., Siegel, B.A., Sobel, B.E., Welch, M.J., Ter-Pogossian, M.M.: Evaluation of myocardial metabolism and perfusion with positron-emitting radionuclides. Progr. Cardiovasc. Dis. 20:191–206, 1977
65. Winbury, M.M.: Experimental studies on the mechanism of

action of nitrates and beta-adrenergic blockers. In: Pharmacologie Clinique des Médicaments Antiangineux, Symposium, Paris, 1974. Basel, Sandoz Editions, 1975, pp. 153–170

66. Wolf, R., Engel, H.J., Hundeshagen, H., Lichtlen, P.: Collateral myocardial blood flow at rest and after maximal arteriolar dilatation in patients with ischemic heart disease. In: Coronary heart Disease, edited by M. Kaltenbach, P. Lichtlen, R. Balcon and W.D. Bussmann. Stuttgart, Thieme, 1978, pp. 61–65
67. Wolf, R., Pretschner, B.P., Engel, H.J., Hundeshagen, H., Lichtlen, P.R.: Effect of Isosorbiddinitrate on ^{201}Thallium myocardial amaging in coronary heart disease (abstract). Am. J. Cardiol. 43:432, 1979
68. Wolfson, W., Heinle, R.A., Herman, M.V., Kemp, H.G., Sullivan, J.M., Gorlin, R.: Propranolol and angina pectoris. Am. J. Cardiol. 18:346–353, 1966
69. Wyatt, H.L., Forrester, J.S., Tyberg, J.V., Goldner, S., Logan, S.E., Parmley, W.W., Swan, H.J.C.: Effect of graded reductions in regional coronary perfusion on regional and total cardiac function. Am. J. Cardiol. 36:185–192, 1975
70. Zierler, K.L.: Equations for measuring blood flow by external monitoring of radioisotopes. Circ. Res. 16:309–321, 1965

Emission Tomography of the Heart: Principles and Applications

J.S. Zielonka and B.L. Holman
Joint Program in Nuclear Medicine, Department of Radiology, Harvard Medical School,
Peter Bent Brigham Hospital, Boston, Massachusetts, USA

Radionuclide methods for evaluation of myocardial ischemia [42, 88] and infarction [42, 43] have become widely available. In addition to providing diagnostic information, these techniques also have predictive value [45]. The accurate interpretation of myocardial scintigraphy is, however, complicated by the compression of a three-dimensional radiopharmaceutical distribution into a two-dimensional image by the detector system. This can cause masking of abnormalities by normal underlying or overlying areas, as well as introduce errors due to superposition of extracardiac activity.

Tomography has shown promise in excluding extracardiac uptake, as well as localizing and quantifying the extent of infarcted or ischemic areas. Because of the wide variety of radiopharmaceuticals, imaging devices, and reconstruction algorithms employed, a review of the tools and principles of radionuclide tomography is presented here.

Imaging Systems

In previous papers, the classification of tomographic systems has been varied to emphasize the particular component of interest. A more general classification, which would include all systems currently in use or under development, and which would make more obvious the shared, as well as unique, aspects of a given system, would be highly desirable. Such a classification can be created by recognizing the required sequence in proceeding from an object to its tomographic representation:

Supported in part by USPHS grant HL 17739. Dr. Holman is an Established Investigator of the American Heart Association.

Address reprint requests to: Jason S. Zielonka, M.D., Department of Radiology, Harvard Medical School, 25 Shattuck Street, Boston, MA 02115, USA

1. Depth position encoding and
2. Detection of emission coupled with x–y position encoding to yield
3. Encoded image data, which undergo
4. Attenuation or detector nonuniformity correction, followed by
5. Reconstruction, which results in
6. Tomographic images.

This classification includes both single-photon and positron devices, single and multiple (opposing and ring) detectors, as well as the various collimators and data acquisition and reconstruction techniques described in the literature. If each of the above functions is examined separately, the advantages and limitations of the individual subsystems can be identified and their effects on the complete system noted.

Position-Encoding Devices

Simple Collimators

Tomographic reconstruction requires views encompassing data from multiple directions; whether these views are obtained simultaneously (as with coded apertures or multiple independent pinholes) or sequentially is irrelevant (assuming no significant change in the distribution of radionuclide within the imaged area during the time of imaging). A simple gamma camera, equipped with any standard collimator, can be used to acquire position-encoded views, which can then be reconstructed (using algorithms to be discussed later). Optimization of collimator design for this form of tomography has been studied [58]. This method has been used with a gamma camera modified to permit rotation of a camera around the stationary patient gantry [53–55]. Alternately, the patient can be rotated in front of a stationary detector system [37, 84].

In one study [37, 84] of both emission computed tomography and a prototype transmission computed tomography unit, seven dogs were examined. In one, used as a control, only thoracotomy was performed, while either the left circumflex or the left anterior descending artery was ligated in the other six dogs. Twenty-four hours after surgery, the animals were injected intravenously with technetium-99m-pyrophosphate; two hours later they were killed and transmission tomographic images were obtained. Quantitative infarct sizing was performed using these images and confirmed histopathologically. A tomographic study was found superior to a study consisting of multiple non-tomographic views, especially for small (2–3 g) infarcts. The radionuclide estimate of infarct size correlated well with the histopathologically determined size and was consistently greater than the histopathologic estimate.

In another animal study [54] the effect of physiologic gating in thallium-201 tomography was studied by examining hearts before and after sacrifice of the animals. Images obtained without gating were found to be more accurate than had been previously thought, presumably because the infarcted areas were already hypokinetic. ^{201}Tl imaging was definitely improved by tomography, although image quality remained inferior to that of ^{99m}Tc images, presumably because of the poor imaging characteristics of thallium with gamma cameras.

In a third study from this group [55], 16 dogs underwent thoracotomy and partial occlusion of either the left anterior descending or the left circumflex artery. Following a 48-hour recovery period, six animals were injected intravenously with ^{99m}Tc-pyrophosphate, sacrificed, and imaged; the remaining ten animals were imaged before and after sacrifice to determine the effect of gating on image deterioration. After sacrifice, the hearts were removed, sectioned, and imaged to provide comparison with the tomographic data. Histopathologic correlation was also obtained. The results were similar to those described above: good imaging of infarcts, especially those of small size (2–3 g), with good correlation (ranging from $r=0.83$ to $r=0.88$) between the radionuclide and pathologic estimates of infarct size. The absence of gating again appeared to have minimal effect on the images.

Multisector Collimators

A slight modification of the above system involves the creation of a collimator that sequentially obtains views from different angles without camera motion; this has been accomplished by: (1) mechanizing the collimator so that it rotates [30–32] and (2) creating a multiple-view collimator, separating each of the images [95].

Cardiac tomography with the rotating collimator, while possible, has not been performed. The multiple-view collimator, using pinholes for imaging each view, has been used in association with ^{201}Tl myocardial imaging by one group, which also described an initial trial with a multi-sector parallel-hole collimator that was terminated because of unacceptable image resolution. The pinhole system, using an iterative reconstruction algorithm to create twelve tomographic planes, achieved a resolution of 1.0 cm (full-width, half-maximum [FWHM]) at a plane 12.7 cm from the collimator face (and a depth resolution of 1.5 cm [FWHM] at that distance). While the original reconstruction algorithm required approximately one hour to generate 12 images, modification of the program and the algorithm reduced this to approximately five minutes.

In a preliminary clinical trial, 42 patients underwent stress myocardial scintigraphy with a parallel-hole and a multipinhole collimator. Of 16 individuals with normal coronary arteries, one had an abnormal parallel-hole study and none had abnormal tomographic studies. Of 26 patients with abnormal coronary angiograms (showing greater than 70% stenosis of at least one major coronary artery), 19 had abnormal parallel-hole studies and 24 had abnormal tomographic studies.

Coded Apertures

The coded apertures used in cardiovascular imaging include the multiple pinhole array (often in the form of a nonredundant array [20, 21, 36]) and the Fresnel zone-plate aperture [20, 29, 36, 44]. Mathematically, the reconstruction methods for both apertures are similar [3, 4, 15, 36], although analogue reconstruction methods have also proven quite useful [20, 29, 36, 44].

The mathematics of image formation using a single pinhole are straightforward. Spatial resolution varies inversely, while detection rate varies directly with pinhole diameter. Additional pinholes increase the detection rate, but also position-encode the image. Thus, in a single exposure, data sufficient to reconstruct all tomographic planes are recorded.

If the vector distance between any two pinholes in a multipinhole array occurs only once, the array is said to be nonredundant. This property results in an autocorrelation function which is peaked in the center and uniform elsewhere. Because of this auto-

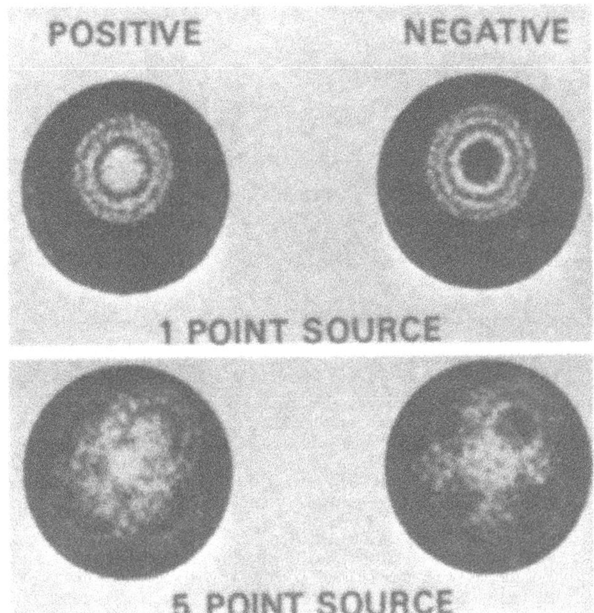

Fig. 1. *Top:* shadowgram produced by a single point source, using a positive (left) and negative (right) Fresnel zone plate. *Bottom:* shadowgram produced using five point sources, demonstrating superposition. (Reprinted with permission from [15]; courtesy of the authors.)

correlation, the same array can then be used to reconstruct an imaged object tomographically. The reconstruction can be performed either mathematically [20] or by analogue techniques [21].

Imaging with multiple pinhole arrays has been limited to demonstrating its feasibility and measuring resolution parameters. No clinical trials of myocardial imaging have been reported.

Fresnel Zone Plate Apertures

With a single pinhole aperture and a point source, an image can be created whose intensity varies with object intensity. When the pinhole is replaced by a Fresnel zone plate, the probability distribution of gamma rays on the image plane is a geometric shadow of the zone plate (Fig. 1). When the point source is replaced by an extended object, the imaging operation is performed by transforming each object point into a zone plate shadow. Since the size of the zone plate shadow varies with the object-aperture distance, three-dimensional position encoding is achieved, with simultaneous data acquisition from all planes.

The reconstruction of a Fresnel shadowgram (as the resulting encoded image is called) is obtained analagously, but results in an image with extremely low contrast, because: (1) an undiffracted component (referred to as "dc light" in optical holography) overlaps a large portion of the image area; and (2) a virtual image is present and superimposed on the true image.

Several methods of overcoming these problems have been described. The first involves using a spatial ing technique to suppress the undiffracted component [1]. Unfortunately, this method results in significant loss of true data, since objects of interest also have low frequency components.

A second analogue method interposes a half-tone screen (Fig. 2) between the object and the zone plate and uses the off-axis portion of the zone plate to encode the image [2, 44]. If certain mathematical criteria are met [2–4], the object spatial frequency spectrum will be passed by the zone plate. The disadvantage of the off-axis zone plate is that it requires a high resolution image detector. Studies have been

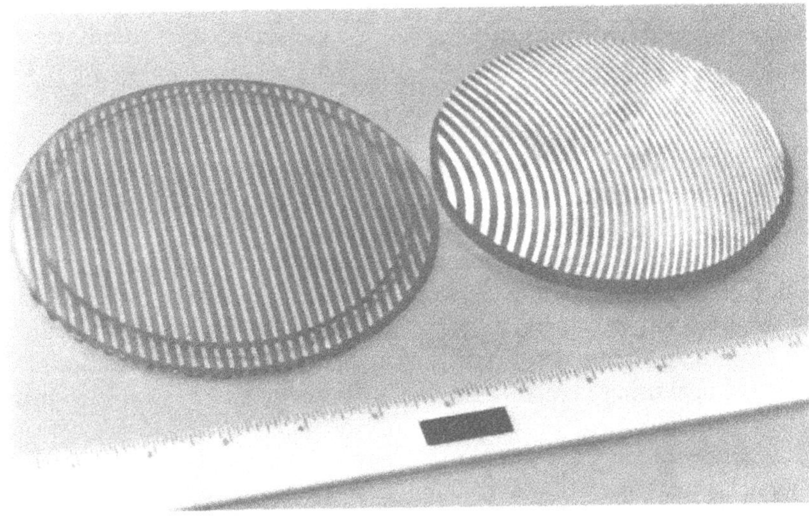

Fig. 2. *Left:* a half-tone screen for use with a Fresnel zone plate. *Right:* the off-axis portion of a Fresnel zone plate.

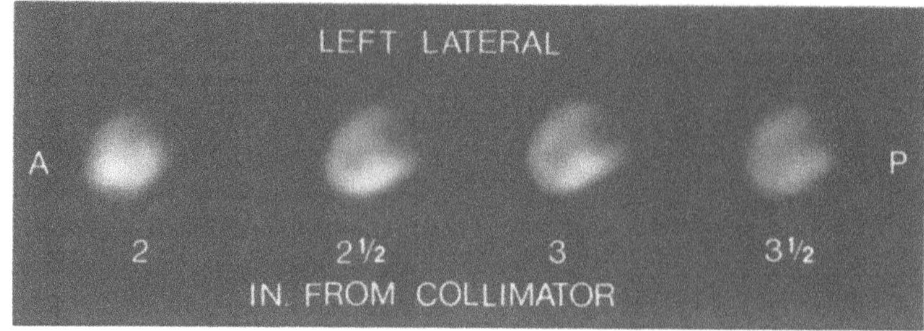

Fig. 3. Tomographic images of a normal canine left ventricle. Note the appearance of the valve plane and the visualization of the ventricular cavity. (Reprinted with permission from [44]; courtesy of the authors.)

performed using (in order of increasing resolution and decreasing sensitivity): Anger-type scintillation cameras [1, 15], image intensifiers [81], multi-wire proportional chambers [67], and radiographic film [2, 29, 44]. Most studies performed using this type of zone plate and an Anger camera have found image quality limited by the spatial resolution of the detector. Radiographic film systems, while maintaining resolution and permitting simple analogue reconstruction, require some photographic manipulation and thus may not be as convenient as a computer-based reconstruction system.

The optical methods described above provide an analogue method for performing Fourier transforms. The zone plate image can also be digitized and reconstructed using computer techniques. This method has been applied with both gamma cameras [15] and multiwire proportional chambers [67].

Cardiac imaging has been performed in animals using an off-axis zone plate system and radiographic film detector. In one study [29], imaging was performed using ^{99m}Tc-macroaggregated albumin (injected into the left atrium) following ligation of the left anterior descending artery. The heart was imaged in vivo both through the open chest and following excision, with good visualization of the cardiac anatomy (Fig. 3) and the infarcted area. In a second study [44], in vivo closed chest imaging after intracoronary injection of ^{99m}Tc-microspheres was performed in normal dogs and in dogs who had had selective coronary artery embolization. Comparison was made to scintillation camera views obtained following sacrifice of the animal. The Fresnel system resolution was 0.64 cm (FWHM). Infarct sizing could not be performed on the scintillation camera views; when the infarct size as measured on the Fresnel system was compared to sizings using in vitro assay methods, the mean error was 13.6%.

While imaging in humans has been performed with Fresnel zone plate apertures (primarily thyroid, lung and bone [29]), no cardiac studies have been reported.

Detector Systems

Single Photon Detectors (Simple Scintillation Detectors)

The simple collimator and standard scintillation camera, as discussed in the previous section, can be specialized for tomographic imaging by creating an array or bank of detectors to obtain multiple views simultaneously [46]. This system is similar in concept to the array system used for positron imaging [40, 75, 76, 90].

In a human clinical trial [46], ^{201}Tl imaging was performed in six normal subjects and five patients with documented myocardial infarctions (infarct age ranging from three months to four years). Comparison was made to multiple-view conventional ^{201}Tl imaging. The patients with infarcts demonstrated markedly reduced ^{201}Tl uptake on the tomographic images in the areas corresponding to their infarcts; the area of reduced uptake was greater on the tomographic study than on the conventional study. The demarcation between normal and abnormal myocardium was clearly defined on the tomographic image; this was generally not true on the views obtained with conventional methods. Separation of other organs was easily achieved using tomography.

Positron Detectors

Positron-emitting radiopharmaceuticals can be used to examine myocardial perfusion, metabolism, and necrosis. Numerous positron-emitting radionuclides have been examined for myocardial imaging, including gallium-68 [17]; rubidium-81 and 82 [16, 48, 99, 101]; ammonia-13 [16, 47]; various compounds using oxygen-15, fluorine-18 [77, 94], and carbon-11; and newer agents [66]. The literature on the classification and physical properties of these compounds has been extensively reviewed elsewhere [98]. Reviews of the physical principles of positron imaging [40, 41, 75,

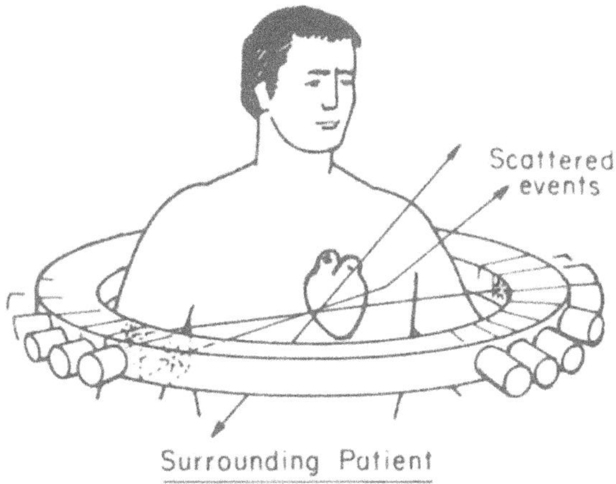

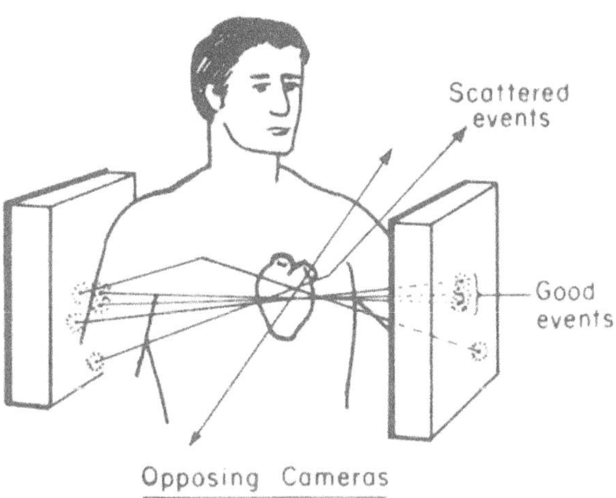

Fig. 4. *Top:* an illustration of the concept of a ring detector; this is also applicable to array detector schemes. *Bottom:* an illustration of opposed detector schemes. (Reprinted with permission; courtesy of T.F. Budinger and F. Rollo.)

76, 90, 93], and of animal and human studies [18, 87] have also been published.

Positron systems can be classified as follows (see Fig. 4 for illustrations of these systems):

1. Two opposed Anger-type scintillation cameras [68];

2. Two opposed multiwire proportional chambers [38, 65];

3. Two opposed planar multicrystal arrays [10, 11, 19];

4. Arrays of opposed crystals [40, 75, 76, 90, 93]; and

5. Rings (multicrystal detectors) [22, 23, 25–27, 80].

The detector properties of the first three systems are similar to those of a single detector of the same type; the last two detector forms are an extension of the dual (opposed) detector concept, allowing multiple coincidence detection and resulting in better spatial resolution and faster reconstruction capabilities. The last two systems are designed for tomography; the first three can be modified to obtain multiple views for subsequent reconstruction.

Work using $^{13}NH_3$ has been reported recently [35, 82], but the radiopharmaceutical used most extensively in animal and human studies to date is a free fatty acid, palmitate, tagged with ^{11}C. The role of free fatty acids in myocardial intermediary metabolism, as well as the effect of ischemia or necrosis on free fatty acid metabolism, has been studied in detail; this provides a strong physiologic foundation for interpretation of ^{11}C-palmitate scans. Studies have been performed in isolated perfused hearts, intact dogs (both normal and with infarctions), and man (both normal individuals and patients with infarctions). In isolated hearts, maintenance of a low-flow state for up to 30 minutes resulted in reversible evidence of ischemia. In dogs, when hypoperfusion was maintained for more than 30 minutes, reperfusion resulted in enhanced accumulation of ^{11}C-palmitate but when hypoperfusion was maintained for more than 60 minutes, ^{11}C-palmitate extraction was permanently diminished. These studies suggest that tomographic evaluation of reversible and irreversible effects of ischemia is possible.

The dog model was also successfully used to study infarction imaging with ^{14}C- and ^{11}C-palmitate, with correlation with enzymatic and histopathologic measures of infarction [93, 97, 98].

Tomographic imaging has now been performed in normal individuals and in patients [86, 87] who, by several clinical measures, had sustained myocardial infarctions. Again, evidence of decreased accumulation of the free fatty acid substrate was seen in anatomic areas corresponding to the clinically determined infarction site. While the number of patients studied to date has been small, the method has clearly been proven in animal studies; the primary limitations to greater use currently are the lack of readily accessible cyclotrons and the limited availability and high cost of tomographic scanning units.

Multiwire Proportional Chambers

The multiwire proportional chamber was developed as a position-sensitive detector for use in particle research. Its potential in nuclear medicine was soon recognized and development undertaken by several groups [5, 64, 65, 74]. Recent reviews have summarized new developments in multiwire proportional chambers [5, 51] and in nuclear medicine applications, in particular [74].

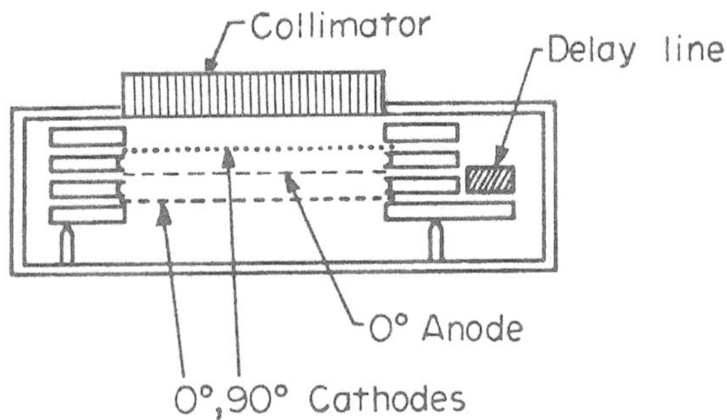

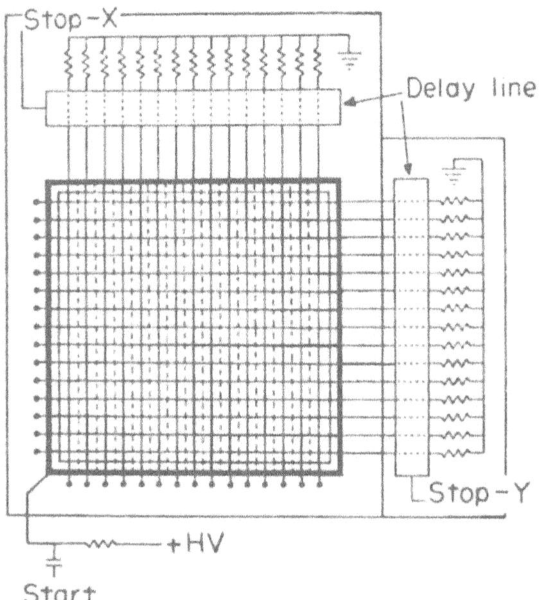

Fig. 5. A schematic diagram of a multiwire proportional chamber, as seen from the side (*top*) and from above (*bottom*). (Reprinted with permission from [73]; courtesy of the author.)

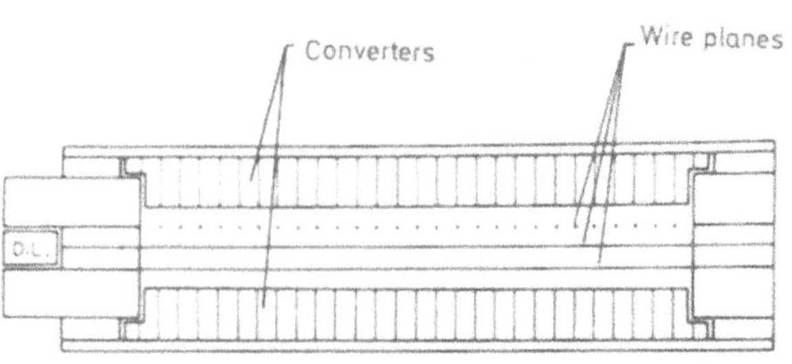

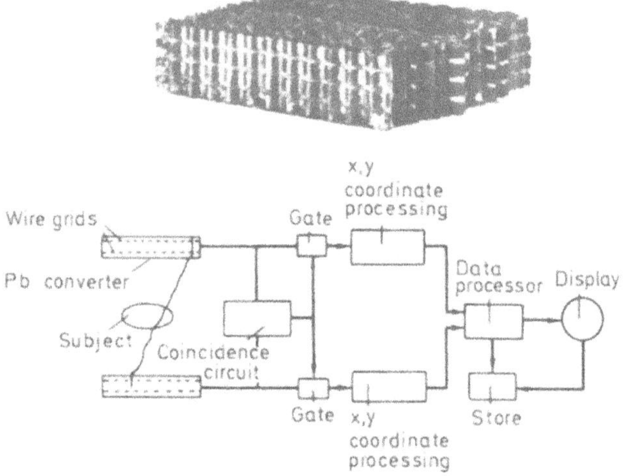

Fig. 6. Two opposed multiwire proportional counters, used for positron imaging and tomography. Note the presence of lead converters, as discussed in the text. *Top:* a view from the side of a single multiwire proportional chamber. *Middle:* a photo of a single multiwire proportional chamber. *Bottom:* a schematic diagram showing the opposed detectors and the subject (left), the coincidence circuits and gates (for positron detection) and the remainder of the data processing equipment (right). (Reprinted with permission from [73]; courtesy of the author.)

While multiwire proportional chambers are most efficient when imaging low-energy (60 keV) gamma rays, units designed for ^{99m}Tc [5], and for positron annihilation energies [21, 64, 65] have been built. The basic multiwire proportional chamber design (Figs. 5 and 6) consists of three parallel planes containing grids of parallel wires, with the wires in the middle plane interconnected and running orthogonally to the other grids. The entire set of grids is placed in a gas-tight envelope, which is filled with some medium (either gas or liquid). The central grid is held at a high positive potential relative to the other grids; this anode grid, on which avalanche multiplication will occur, provides pulse-height data on the incoming photon, while the two outer cathode grids provide spatial information about it.

A photon entering the chamber interacts with the surrounding gaseous (or liquid) medium by the photoelectric effect. The resulting photoelectron creates secondary electrons (within a small volume) by ionization. These electrons drift within the electric field towards the anode, where, after avalanche multiplication, an amplified pulse is produced with an amplitude proportional to the energy of the photoelectron. The spatial coordinates of the event can be deduced from a simultaneous pulse produced on the cathode wires.

In any practical system, the characteristics of the detector are determined by design compromises involving several important parameters. Certain characteristics, however, depend strongly on single factors and, for multiwire proportional chambers, spatial resolution is determined by the cathode interwire and cathode-cathode spacing, as well as by the density of the surrounding gaseous or liquid medium; one of the disadvantages of multiwire proportional chambers for clinical nuclear medicine is the requirement of some systems for maintaining this medium

Table 1. Conversion efficiency and resolution of several multiwire proportional chambers for energies of clinical interest

Energy source	Gamma energy (keV)	Conversion (%)	Resolution (mm, FWHM)	Ref.
^{201}Tl	69–83[a]	–	1.7	[73]
^{178}Ta	54–64	–	2.5	[73]
^{99m}Tc	140	15	3	[5]
Positron emitters	511	2.5	6	[74]

[a] Measurements made primarily at 35 keV, the dominant photoelectron energy

at several atmospheres' pressure. The event counting rate is determined by the readout capacity of the electronics used; with current technology, rates of approximately 10^5 events/sec should be possible. The detection efficiency is a complex function [5], but for a given configuration, it decreases as the energy of the incident photon increases. Currently achieved conversion efficiency and spatial resolution are given in Table 1.

For single-photon imaging, true system resolution is thus dependent on the type of collimator used; it has been suggested that the coded aperture, in conjunction with a low-energy gamma emitter (such as tantalum-178) and a multiwire proportional chamber detector, would be extremely effective [45, 70, 74].

In order to improve conversion efficiency in positron imaging, a lead collimator is used. Although this results in a loss of pulse-height data (Fig. 6), this is of little significance in this form of imaging.

Other Detectors

Image Intensifiers

The use of image intensifier cameras for clinical cardiovascular imaging has not yet been extensively reported [49, 63, 69], although this system has been used (in conjunction with a Fresnel zone plate [81]) in a configuration permitting tomography [57, 63].

Semiconductor Cameras

Instead of converting an incoming photon into a scintillation, as does the Anger-type scintillation camera, a semiconductor camera converts the photon into an electrical signal. This type of device has significantly better energy resolution than does the scintillation camera, permitting electronic exclusion of scatter. The superior energy resolution of the semiconductor camera can also be used to achieve some statistical enhancement in detection of "hot spots" against background activity [78].

While the semiconductor camera offers some advantages for cardiac studies, such as simultaneous multiple tracer techniques, no clinical studies have been reported to date.

Reconstruction Methods

The problem of reconstructing a three-dimensional distribution, given an externally mapped density distribution, is not a new one; extensive mathematical analysis of this problem was performed by Radon [79] in 1917. Nor is the problem uniquely of interest to nuclear medicine; early solutions were required to determine the distribution of solar microwave radiation [6–8], the spatial structure of complex biomolecules from their electron micrographs [28], and certain problems in optics and acoustic transmission. For medical applications, certain investigators in nuclear medicine and radiology [60–62] developed reconstruction tomographic techniques as an improvement on the well-known technique of longitudinal radiographic (blurring) tomography; in 1972, Hounsfield coupled these techniques with a high-speed digital computer, a gantry system, and a highly collimated source, thus introducing transmission computerized tomography [50].

While the reconstruction methods for transmission and emission computed tomography are identical mathematically, there are several fundamental differences in sources of data and corrections required. These have been discussed elsewhere [24, 92] and will only be summarized here:

1. In transmission computed tomography the variable measured (which provides the profiles used in reconstruction) is the attenuation of the x-ray beam through the traversed tissue; in emission computed tomography the variable measured is the distribution of activity within the tissue, as altered by attenuation (which varies with the radionuclide and the tissue);

2. In transmission computed tomography attenuation is essentially independent of tissue depth; in emission computed tomography this is true for systems that use annihilation-coincidence detection, but not for single-photon imaging systems;

3. In transmission computed tomography resolution and field of view are independent of tissue depth, while this is not true for emission computed tomography.

The number of events is less with emission than with transmission computed tomography, resulting

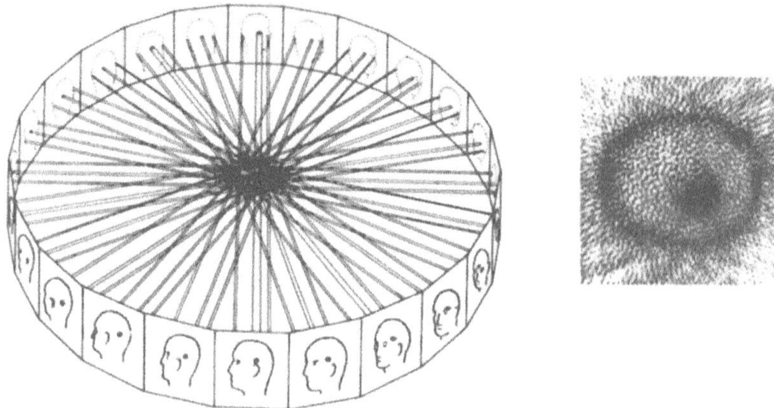

Fig. 7. An illustration of the basic concept of reconstruction tomography: by taking data from multiple two-dimensional views (taken at slightly different angles) and back-projecting, a three-dimensional distribution of activity in the subject can be obtained. *Right*: a detailed view of the reconstructed image, showing the contribution of each projection to the final image. (Reprinted with permission from [92]; courtesy of the author.)

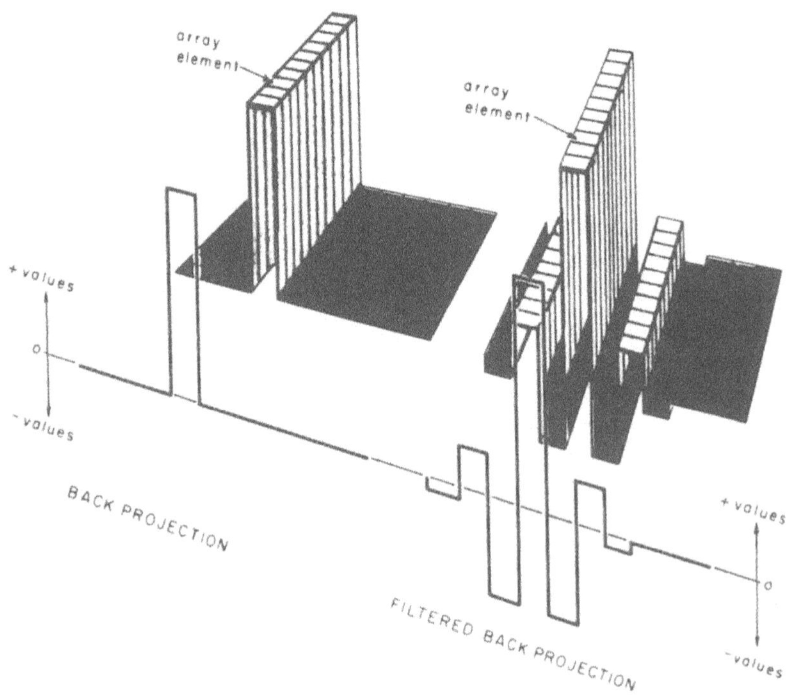

Fig. 8. *Left:* In the back-projection method, the value assigned to a given array element is the ray-sum; no correction is made at this stage for surrounding activity – hence, the resulting "star artifacts." *Right:* In the filtered back-projection method, the value assigned to a given array element also affects the value assigned to neighboring array elements; this tends to correct the "star artifact." (Reprinted with permission from [92]; courtesy of the author.)

in poorer statistics, but offsetting this disadvantage somewhat is the increased object contrast provided by emission computed tomography.

Several mathematical reviews of reconstruction techniques, of various degrees of rigor [13, 14, 33, 39, 96] and readability [9, 18, 34, 56, 84, 92], are now available; the reader is referred to them for details beyond those included in this section, which will, in a qualitative fashion, classify and describe the currently used reconstruction methods and note some of their advantages and disadvantages.

Back-Projection (Figs. 7 and 8)

Back-projection is the simplest reconstruction method and was the first devised; it has been replaced in current systems with more advanced techniques. It is discussed here for conceptual reasons.

In back-projection, reconstruction is performed by assigning the value of the ray-sum to each element of the ray. Since the back-projected density at each point is the sum of all ray-sums passing through the point, this method is sometimes referred to as the summation method.

The prime limitation of this method is the introduction of "star artifacts" corresponding to poor reconstruction of discrete areas of increased density; this is an inherent defect in the algorithm.

Iterative Reconstruction

The mathematical analysis of the reconstruction problem results in closed solutions for an infinite number of measurement angles and for a minimal beam width. If the practical approximations of finite beam width and a finite number of measuring angles are made, the problem becomes one of solving a (large) set of simultaneous algebraic equations. While the direct mathematical method (matrix inversion) can be used, several other techniques have been developed that apply corrections to the measured cell densities to approximate the measured ray-projections more closely. After a correction algorithm has been applied to all data, the process is repeated (hence the name iterative) until the desired degree of accuracy has been obtained. In each algorithm the correction may be applied as an additive or as a multiplicative correction.

Simultaneous Correction (ILST) [7, 8, 12, 13]

With simultaneous correction, all the ray sums are calculated first, with the corrections applied to all the cells simultaneously. The next iteration is then performed. It can be shown mathematically that this method as described does not converge to a solution; a damping factor is required, the exact form of which is not critical. Since one of the original damping factors was chosen to achieve the best least-squares fit to the data, this method is also called iterative least squares technique (ILST).

Point-by-Point Correction (SIRT)

For point-by-point correction, all the ray-sums through a given point are first calculated and the total correction is then applied to that point. This process is then repeated for the remaining points in the matrix.

While this process converges without needing a damping factor, it requires more arithmetic processing per iteration than does simultaneous correction. This method is also called the simultaneous iterative reconstruction technique (SIRT).

Ray-by-Ray Correction (ART)

Ray-by-ray correction was the method originally used by Hounsfield [50], as well as by Kuhl and Edwards [59–62]. The method is also called the arithmetic reconstruction technique (ART). This technique is more efficient than the other iterative procedures; however, it is also more sensitive to noisy data.

Analytic Reconstruction Techniques

Rather than performing a series of approximations towards a solution, it is possible to attempt a direct solution to the equation relating the observed emission density and the three-dimensional distribution. In order to be implemented with digital techniques, this method requires spatial resolution (i.e., bandwidth) limitation. While the most frequent methods used involve Fourier series, more complex solutions have been considered [83].

Two-Dimensional Fourier Reconstruction

A straightforward solution of the mathematical equations of reconstruction can be achieved by two-dimensional Fourier reconstruction; in this method rapid calculation algorithms are used to achieve acceptable reconstruction times. Certain investigators, using optical methods, have, in essence, performed an analogue reconstruction in this manner also.

Filtered Back-Projection (Figs. 7 and 8)

If a more accurate ray-sum profile is used in the simple back-projection algorithm previously described, a solution similar to that obtained from the equations describing two-dimensional Fourier reconstruction results. This is the basis of filtered back-projection. The type of filtration applied to the ray-sum profile can be one of the three varieties listed above; at the present time, convolutional filtering is most commonly used in commercial transmission computed tomography devices.

Comparison

The reconstruction methods currently in use for both transmission and emission computed tomography units have been described in the literature [9]; emission tomographic systems use filtered back-projection or an iterative method almost exclusively. The comparison of analytic and iterative methods is complex, involving considerations of resolution, speed of reconstruction, and cost of equipment. Studies to determine better measures of algorithm efficiency and accuracy are being performed [37, 72, 85, 96, 100].

Comparison of tomography performed with single-photon and positron agents on phantoms is now being made [17]. The results seem to indicate better resolution with positron imaging, at the cost of increased equipment and support (i.e., cyclotron) services.

References

1. Barrett, H.H.: Fresnel zone plate imaging in nuclear medicine. J. Nucl. Med. 13:382–385, 1972

2. Barrett, H.H., Wilson, D.T., DeMeester, G.D.: The use of half-tone screens in Fresnel zone plate imaging or incoherent sources. Optics Commun. 5:398–401, 1972
3. Barrett, H.H., Horrigan, F.A.: Fresnel zone plate imaging of gamma rays; theory. Appl. Optics 12:2686–2702, 1973
4. Barrett, H.H., DeMeester, G.D., Wilson, D.T., Farmelant, M.H.: Tomographic imaging with a Fresnel zone plate system. In: Tomographic Imaging in Nuclear Medicine, edited by G.S. Freedman. New York, Society of Nuclear Medicine, 1973, pp. 106–120
5. Bateman, J.E., Connolly, J.F.: A multiwire proportional gamma camera for imaging ^{99m}Tc radionuclide. Phys. Med. Biol. 23:455–470, 1978
6. Bracewell, R.N.: Two dimensional aerial smoothing in radio astronomy. Austral. J. Phys. 9:297–314, 1956
7. Bracewell, R.N.: Strip integration in radio astronomy. Austral. J. Phys. 9:197, 1956
8. Bracewell, R.N., Riddle, A.C.: Inversion of fanbeam scans in radio astronomy. Astrophys. J. 150:427–434, 1967
9. Brooks, R.A., DiChiro, G.: Principles of computer assisted tomography (CAT) in radiographic and radioisotopic imaging. Phys. Med. Biol. 21:689–732, 1976
10. Brownell, G.L., Burnham, C.A.: The MGH positron camera. In: Tomographic imaging in Nuclear Medicine, edited by G.S. Freedman. New York, Society of Nuclear Medicine, 1973, pp. 154–164
11. Brownell, G.L., Burnham, C.A., Chesler, D.A., Correia, J.A., Correll, J.E., Hoop, B., Parker, J.A., Subramanyam, R.: Transverse section imaging of radionuclide distributions in heart, lung and brain. In: Reconstruction Tomography in Diagnostic Radiology and Nuclear Medicine, edited by M.M. Ter-Pogossian, M.E. Phelps, G.L. Brownell, J.R. Cox, D.O. Davis, R.G. Evens. Baltimore, University Park Press, 1977, pp. 293–307
12. Budinger, T.F., Gullberg, G.T.: Three dimensions in reconstruction in nuclear medicine by iterative least squares and Fourier transform techniques. Lawrence Berkely Lab Report no. LBL-2146, 1974
13. Budinger, T.F., Gullberg, G.T.: Three dimensional reconstruction in nuclear medicine by iterative least squares and Fourier transform techniques. IEEE Trans. Nucl. Sci. NS-21:2–20, 1974
14. Budinger, T.F., Gullberg, G.T : Three dimensional reconstruction of isotope distributions. Phys. Med. Biol. 19:378–380, 1974
15. Budinger, T.F., McDonald, R.: Reconstruction of the Fresnel-coded gamma camera images by digital computer. J. Nucl. Med. 16:309–313, 1975
16. Budinger, T.F., Yano, Y., Hoop, B.: A comparison of $^{82}Rb^{+}$ and $^{13}NH_3$ for myocardial positron scintigraphy. J. Nucl. Med. 16:429–431, 1975
17. Budinger, T.F., Derenzo, S.E., Gullberg, G.T., Greenberg, W.L., Huesman, R.H.: Emission computer assisted tomography with single-photon and positron annihilation photon emitters. J. Comput. Assist. Tomog. 1:131–145, 1977
18. Budinger, T.F., Gullberg, G.T.: Transverse section reconstruction of gamma-ray emitting radionuclides in patients. In: Reconstruction Tomography in Diagnostic Radiology and Nuclear Medicine, edited by M.M. Ter-Pogossian, M.E. Phelps, G.L. Brownell, J.R. Cox, D.O. Davis, R.G. Evens. Baltimore, University Park Press, 1977, pp. 315–342
19. Burnham, C.A., Brownell, G.L.: A multicrystal positron camera. IEEE Trans. Nucl. Sci NS-19:201–205, 1973
20. Chang, L.T., Kaplan, S.N., MacDonald, B., Perez-Mendez, V., Shiraishi, L.: A method of tomographic imaging using a multiple pinhole-coded aperture. J. Nucl. Med. 15:1063–1065, 1974
21. Chang, L.T., MacDonald, B., Perez-Mendez, V.: Axial tomography and three-dimensional image reconstruction. IEEE Trans. Nucl. Sci. NS-23:568–572, 1976
22. Cho, Z.H., Eriksson, L., Chan, J.: A circular ring transverse axial positron camera. In: Reconstruction Tomography in Diagnostic Radiology and Nuclear Medicine, edited by M.M. Ter-Pogossian, M.E. Phelps, G.L. Brownell, J.R. Cox, D.O. Davis, R.G. Evens: Baltimore, University Park Press, 1977, pp. 393–424
23. Cho, Z.H., Cohen, M.B., Singh, M., Eriksson, L., Chan, J., MacDonald, N., Spolter, L.: Performance and evaluation of the circular ring transverse axial positron camera (CRTAPC). IEEE Trans. Nucl. Sci. NS-24:530–543, 1977
24. Depresseux, J.C.: Positron emission tomography and its applications. J. Belg. Rad. 60:483–500, 1977
25. Derenzo, S.E., Zaklad, H., Budinger, T.F.: Analytical study of a high-resolution positron ring detector system for transaxial reconstruction tomography. J. Nucl. Med. 16:1166–1173, 1975
26. Derenzo, S.E.: Positron ring cameras for emission-computed tomography. IEEE Trans. Nucl. Med. NS-24:881–885, 1977
27. Derenzo, S.E., Budinger, T.F., Cahoon, J.L., Huesman, R.H., Jackson, H.G.: High resolution computed tomography of positron emitters. IEEE Trans. Nucl. Med. NS-24:544–558, 1977
28. Derosier, D.J., Klug, A.: Reconstruction of three-dimensional structure from electron micographs. Nature 217:130, 1968
29. Farmelant, M.A., Demeester, G., Wilson, D., Barrett, H.: Initial clinical experiences with a Fresnel zone-plate imager. J. Nucl. Med. 16:183–187, 1975
30. Freedman, G.S.: Tomography with a gamma camera – theory. J. Nucl. Med. 11:602–604, 1970
31. Freedman, G.S.: Gamma camera tomography – preliminary clinical experience. Radiology 102:365–369, 1972
32. Freedman, G.S.: Digital gamma camera tomography – theory. In: Tomographic Imaging in Nuclear Medicine, edited by G.S. Freedman. New York, Society of Nuclear Medicine, 1973, pp. 68–75
33. Gordon, R., Herman, G.T.: Three dimensional reconstruction from projections: A review of algorithms. Int. Rev. Cytol. 38:111–151, 1974
34. Gordon, R.: A tutorial on ART, algebraic reconstruction techniques. IEEE Trans. Nucl. Sci. NS-21:78–93, 1974
35. Gould, K.L., Schelbert, H.R., Phelps, M.E., Hoffmann, E.J.: Noninvasive assessment of coronary stenoses with myocardial perfusion imaging during pharmacologic coronary vasodilatation. V. Detection of 47 percent diameter coronary stenosis with intravenous nitrogen-13 ammonia and emission-computed tomography in intact dogs. Am. J. Cardiol. 43:200–208, 1979
36. Groh, G., Hayat, G.S., Stroke, G.W.: X-ray and gamma-ray imaging with multiple pinhole cameras using a posteriori image synthesis. Appl. Optics 11:191–193, 1972
37. Gustafson, D.E., Singh, M., Berggren, M.J., Dewanjee, M.K., Bahn, R.C., Ritman, E.L.: Emission computed tomography – application to acute myocardial infarct imaging in intact dogs using Tc-99m pyrophosphate (abstract). J. Nucl. Med. 19:684, 1978
38. Hattner, R.S., Lim, C.B., Swann, S.J., Kaufman, L., Perez-Mendez, V., Chu, D., Huberty, J.P., Price, D.C., Wilson, C.B.: Cerebral imaging using ^{68}Ga-DTPA and the UCSF multi-wire proportional chamber positron camera. IEEE Nucl. Sci. NS-23:523–525, 1976
39. Herman, G.T., Hurwitz, H., Jr., Lent, A.: A Bayesian analysis of image reconstruction. In: Reconstruction Tomography in Diagnostic Radiology and Nuclear Medicine, edited by M.M. Ter-Pogossian, M.E. Phelps, G.L. Brownell, J.R. Cox, D.O. Davis, R.G. Evens. Baltimore, University Park Press, 1977, pp. 85–104

40. Hoffman, E.J., Phelps, M.E., Mullani, N.A., Higgins, C.S., Ter-Pogossian, M.M.: Design and performance characteristics of a whole body positron transaxial tomograph. J. Nucl. Med. 17:493–502, 1976
41. Hoffman, E.J., Phelps, M.E.: An analysis of some of the physical aspects of positron transaxial tomography. Comput. Biol. Med. 6:345–360, 1976
42. Holman, B.L.: Radionuclide methods in the evaluation of myocardial ischemia and infarction. Circulation (Suppl.) 53:I-112–119, 1976
43. Holman, B.L., Davis, M.A., Hanson, R.N.: Myocardial infarct imaging with technetium-labelled complexes. Sem. Nucl. Med. 7:29–35, 1977
44. Holman, B.L., Idoine, J.D., Sos, T.A., Tancrell, R., DeMeester, G.: Tomographic scintigraphy of regional myocardial perfusion. J. Nucl. Med. 18:764–769, 1977
45. Holman, B.L., Harris, G.I., Neirinckx, R.D., Jones, A.G., Idoine, T.: Tantalum-178 – a short-lived radionuclide for nuclear medicine: Production of the parent W-178. J. Nucl. Med. 19:510–513, 1978
46. Holman, B.L., Hill, T.C., Wynne, J., Lovett, R.D., Smith, E.M.: Single photon transaxial emission computed tomography of the heart in normal subjects and in patients with infarction. J. Nucl. Med. (in press)
47. Hoop, B. Jr., Smith, T.W., Burnham, C.A., Correll, J.E., Brownell, G.L., Sanders, C.A.: Myocardial imaging by means of $^{13}NH4^{+}$ and multicrystal positron camera. J. Nucl. Med. 14:181–183, 1973
48. Hoop, B., Beh, R.A., Beller, G.A., Brownell, G.L., Burnham, C.A., Hnatowich, D.J., Moore, R.H., Parker, J.A., Roux-Lough, P.O., Smith, T.W., Budinger, T.F., Chu, P., Yano, Y., Barnes, J.W., Grant, P.M., Ogard, A.E., O'Brien, H.A.: Myocardial positron scintigraphy with short-lived 82-Rb. IEEE Trans. Nucl. Sci. NS-23:584–589, 1976
49. Horowitz, N.H., Lofstron, I.E., Forsaith, A.L.: The Spintharicon: A new approach to radiation imaging. J. Nucl. Med. 6:724–739, 1965
50. Hounsfield, G.N.: Computerized transverse axial scanning (tomography): Part 1: description of system. Br. J. Radiol. 46:1016–1022, 1973
51. Jeavons, A.P., Charpak, G., Stubbs, R.J.: The high-density multiwire drift chamber. Nucl. Instrum. Meth. 124:491–503, 1975
52. Kaufman, L., Perez-Mendez, V., Rindi, A., Sperinde, J.M., Wollenberg, H.A.: Wire spark chambers for clinical imaging of gamma-rays. Phys. Med. Biol. 16:417–426, 1971
53. Keyes, J.W., Jr., Orlandea, N., Heetderks, W.J., Leonard, P.F., Rogers, W.L.: The Humungotron – a scintillation camera transaxial tomograph. J. Nucl. Med. 18:381–387, 1977
54. Keyes, J.W., Leonard, P.F., Svethoff, D.J., Brody, S.L., Rogers, W.L., Lucchesi, B.R.: Myocardial imaging using emission computed tomography. Radiology 127:809–812, 1978
55. Keyes, J.W., Leonard, P.F., Brody, S.L., Svetkoff, D.J., Rogers, L., Lucchesi, B.R.: Myocardial infarct quantification in dog by single photon emission computed tomography. Circulation 58:227–232, 1978
56. Keyes, W.I.: A practical approach to transverse-section gamma-ray imaging. Br. J. Radiol. 49:62–70, 1976
57. Kirch, D.L., Steele, P.P., LeFree, M.T., Evans, P.L., Stern, D.M., Vogel, R.A.: Application of a computerized image-intensifier radionuclide imaging system to the study of regional left ventricular dysfunction. IEEE Trans. Nucl. Sci. NS-23:507–515, 1976
58. Kircos, L.T., Leonard, P.F., Keyes, J.W.: Optimized collimator for single-photon computed tomography with a scintillation camera. J. Nucl. Med. 19:322–323, 1978
59. Kuhl, D.E., Edwards, R.Q., Ricci, A.R., Reivich, M.: Quantitative section scanning using orthogonal tangent correction. J. Nucl. Med. 14:196–200, 1973
60. Kuhl, D.E., Edwards, R.A.: Image separation in radioisotope scanning. Radiology 80:653–662, 1963
61. Kuhl, D.E., Hale, J., Eaton, W.L.: Transmission scanning: A useful adjunct to conventional emission scanning for accurately keying isotope deposition to radiographic anatomy. Radiology 87:278–284, 1966
62. Kuhl, D.E., Edwards, R.Q.: Reorganizing data from transverse section scans using digital processing. Radiology 91:975–983, 1968
63. Lantz, B., Lindberg, B., Huebel, J.: Computerized tomography of human heart by video technique. In: Roentgen-Video-Techniques for Dynamic Studies of Structure and Function of the Heart and Circulation, edited by P.H. Heintzen, J.H. Bursch. Stuttgart, Thieme, 1978, pp. 328–335
64. Lim, C.B., Chu, D., Kaufman, L., Perez-Mendez, V., Sperinde, J.: Characteristics of multiwire proportional chambers for positron imaging. IEEE Trans. Nucl. Sci. NS-21:85–88, 1974
65. Lim, C.B., Chu, D., Kaufman, L., Perez-Mendez, V., Hattner, R., Price, D.: Initial characterization of a multi-wire proportional chamber positron camera. IEEE Trans. Nucl. Sci. NS-22:388–394, 1975
66. Machulla, H.J., Stocklin, G., Kupfernagel, C., Freundlieb, C., Höck, A., Vyksa, K., Feinendegen, L.E.: Comparative evaluation of fatty acids labelled with C-11, Cl-34m, Br-77, and I-123 for metabolic studies of the myocardium: Concise communication. J. Nucl. Med. 19:298–302, 1978
67. MacDonald, B., Chang, G.T., Perez-Mendez, V., Shiraishi, L.: Gamma-ray imaging using a Fresnel-zone plate aperture, multiwire proportional counter detector and computer reconstruction. IEEE Trans. Nucl. Sci. NS-21:678–684, 1974
68. Muehllehner, O.: Performance parameters for a tomographic scintillation camera. In: Tomographic Imaging in Nuclear Medicine, edited by G.S. Freedman. New York, Society of Nuclear Medicine, 1973, pp. 76–82
69. Mulder, H., Pauwels, E.K.J.: A new nuclear medicine scintillation camera based on image intensifier tubes. J. Nucl. Med. 17:1008–1012, 1976
70. Neirinckx, R.D., Jones, A.G., Davis, M.A., Harris, G.I., Holman, B.L.: Tantalum-178 – a short-lived nuclide for nuclear medicine: Development of a potential generator system. J. Nucl. Med. 19:514–519, 1978
71. Oppenheim, B.E., Harper, P.V.: Iterative three-dimensional reconstruction: A search for a better algorithm. J. Nucl. Med. 15:520, 1974
72. Oppenheim, B.E.: Reconstructive tomography from incomplete projections. In: Reconstruction Tomography in Diagnostic Radiology and Nuclear Medicine, edited by M.M. Ter-Pogossian, M.E. Phelps, G.L. Brownell, J.R. Cox, D.O. Davis, R.G. Evens. Baltimore, University Park Press, 1977, pp. 155–184
73. Parsignault, D.R., Gorenstein, P., Zimmerman, R.E., Burns, R.: Radioisotope imaging with a xenon-filled multiwire proportional counter. IEEE Trans. Nucl. Sci. NS-26:563–564, 1979
74. Perez-Mendez, V., Kaufman, L., Lim, C.B., Price, D.C., Blumin, L., Cavalieri, R.: Multiwire proportional chambers in nuclear medicine: Present status and perspectives. Int. J. Nucl. Med. Biol. 3:29–33, 1976
75. Phelps, M.E., Hoffman, E.J., Mullani, N.A., Ter-Pogossian, M.M.: Application of annhilation coincidence detection to trans-axial reconstruction tomography. J. Nucl. Med. 16:210–224, 1975
76. Phelps, M.E., Hoffman, E.J., Huang, S.C., Kuhl, D.E.: ECAT: A new computerized tomographic imaging system for

positron-emitting radiopharmaceuticals. J. Nucl. Med. 19:635–647, 1978

77. Phelps, M.E., Hoffman, E.J., Selin, C., Huang, S.C., Robinson, G., MacDonald, N., Schelbert, H., Kuhl, D.E.: Investigation of [^{18}F]2-fluoro-2-deoxyglucose for the measure of myocardial glucose metabolism. J. Nucl. Med. 19:1311–1319, 1978
78. Profio, A.E., Cho, Z.H.: Semiconductor camera for detection of small tumors. J. Nucl. Med. 16:53–57, 1975
79. Radon, J.: Über die Bestimmung von Funktionen durch ihre Integralwerte längs gewisser Mannigfaltigkeiten. Ber. Verk. Sach. Akad. 69:262–277, 1917
80. Robertson, J.S., Marr, R.B., Rosenblum, B., Radeka, V., Yamamoto, Y.L.: 32 crystal positron transverse section detector. In: Tomographic Imaging in Nuclear Medicine, edited by G.S. Freedman. New York, Society of Nuclear Medicine, 1973, pp. 142–153
81. Rogers, W.L., Han, KS., Jones, L.W., Beierwaltes, W.H.: Application of a Fresnel zone plate to gamma-ray imaging. J. Nucl. Med. 13:612–615, 1972
82. Schelbert, H.R., Phelps, M.E., Hoffman, E.J., Huang, S.C., Selin, C.E., Kuhl, D.E.: Regional myocardial perfusion assessed with ^{13}N labelled ammonia and positron emission computerized axial tomography. Am. J. Cardiol. 43:209–218, 1979
83. Shepp, L.A., Kruskal, J.B.: Computerized tomography: The new medical x-ray technology. Am. Math. Monthly 85:420–439, 1978
84. Singh, M., Berggren, M.J., Gustafson, D.E., Dewanjee, M.K., Bahn, R.C., Ritman, E.L.: Emission computed tomography and its application to imaging of acute myocardial infarction in intact dogs using Tc-99m pyrophosphate. J. Nucl. Med. 20:50–56, 1979
85. Snyder, D.L., Cox, J.R., Jr.: An overview of reconstructive tomography and limitations imposed by a finite number of projections. In: Reconstruction Tomography in Diagnostic Radiology and Nuclear Medicine, edited by M.M. Ter-Pogossian, M.E. Phelps, G.L. Brownell, J.R. Cox, D.O. Davis, R.G. Evens. Baltimore, University Park Press, 1977, pp. 3–32
86. Sobel, B.E., Weiss, E.S., Welch, M.J., Siegel, B., Ter-Pogossian, M.M.: Detection of remote myocardial infarction in patients with positron emission transaxial tomography and intravenous ^{11}C-palmitate. Circulation 55:853–857, 1977
87. Sobel, B.E.: External quantification of myocardial ischemia and infarction with positron-emitting radionuclides. Adv. Cardiol. 22:29–47, 1978
88. Strauss, H.W., Harrison, K., Langan, J.K., Lebowitz, E., Pitt, B.: Thallium-201 for myocardial imaging: Relation of thallium-201 to regional myocardial perfusion. Circulation 51:641–645, 1975
89. Ter-Pogossian, M.M., Niklas, W.F., Ball, J., Eichling, J.O.: An image scintillation camera for use with radioactive isotopes emitting low energy photons. Radiology 86:463–469, 1966
90. Ter-Pogossian, M.M., Phelps, M.E., Hoffman, E.S., Mullani, N.A.: A positron emission transaxial tomograph for nuclear medicine imaging (PETT). Radiology 114:89–98, 1975
91. Ter-Pogossian, M.M., Hoffman, E.J., Weiss, E.S.: Positron emission reconstruction tomography for the assessment of regional myocardial metabolism by the administration of substrates labelled with cyclotron-produced radionuclides. In: Conference on Cardiovascular Imaging and Image Processing: Ultrasound, Angiography and Isotopes. Stanford University (Stanford, CA), 1975
92. Ter-Pogossian, M.M.: Basic principles of computed axial tomography. Sem. Nucl. Med. 7:109–127, 1977
93. Ter-Pogossian, M.M., Mullani, N.A., Hood, J., Higgins, C.S., Currie, C.M.: A multislice positron emission computed tomograph (PETT IV) yielding transverse and longitudinal images. Radiology 128:477–484, 1978
94. Tewson, T.J., Welch, M.J., Raichle, M.E.: [^{18}F]-labelled 3-deoxy-3-fluoro-D-glucose: synthesis and preliminary biodistribution data. J. Nucl. Med. 19:1339–1345, 1978
95. Vogel, R.A., Kirch, D., LeFree, M., Steele, P.: A new method of multiplanar emission tomography using a seven pinhole collimator and an Anger scintillation camera. J. Nucl. Med. 19:648–654, 1978
96. Walters, T.E., Simon, W., Chesler, D.A., Correia, J.A.: Iterative convolution for radionuclide axial tomography with correction for internal absorption. In: Reconstruction Tomography in Diagnostic Radiology and Nuclear Medicine, edited by M.M. Ter-Pogossian, M.E. Phelps, G.L. Brownell, J.R. Cox, D.O. Davis, R.G. Evens. Baltimore, University Park Press, 1977, pp. 309–314
97. Weiss, E.S., Ahmed, S.A., Welch, M.J., Williamson, J.R., Ter-Pogossian, M.M., Sobel, B.E.: Quantification of infarction in cross sections of canine myocardium in vivo with positron emission transaxial tomography and ^{11}C-palmitate. Circulation 55:66–73, 1977
98. Weiss, E.S., Siegal, B.A., Sobel, B.E., Welch, M.J., Ter-Pogossian, M.M.: Evaluation of myocardial metabolism and perfusion with positron-emitting radionuclides. In: Principles of Cardiovascular Nuclear Medicine, edited by B.L. Holman, E.H. Sonnenblick, M. Lesch. New York, Grune & Stratton, 1978, pp. 67–82
99. Yano, Y., Anger, H.O.: Visualization of heart and kidneys in animals with ultra-short lived ^{82}Rb and the positron scintillation camera J. Nucl. Med. 9:412–415, 1968
100. Zacher, R.: Resolution limits for reconstructive tomography based on photon attenuation. In: Reconstruction Tomography in Diagnostic Radiology and Nuclear Medicine, edited by M.M. Ter-Pogossian, M.E. Phelps, G.L. Brownell, J.R. Cox, D.O. Davis, R.G. Evens. Baltimore, University Park Press, 1977, pp. 59–66
101. Zaret B.L.: Imaging with potassium and its analogs. In: Principles of Cardiovascular Nuclear Medicine, edited by B.L. Holman, E.H. Sonnenblick, M. Lesch. New York, Grune & Stratton, 1977, pp. 53–66

GPSR Compliance
The European Union's (EU) General Product Safety Regulation (GPSR) is a set of rules that requires consumer products to be safe and our obligations to ensure this.

If you have any concerns about our products, you can contact us on

ProductSafety@springernature.com

In case Publisher is established outside the EU, the EU authorized representative is:

Springer Nature Customer Service Center GmbH
Europaplatz 3
69115 Heidelberg, Germany

www.ingramcontent.com/pod-product-compliance
Ingram Content Group UK Ltd.
Pitfield, Milton Keynes, MK11 3LW, UK
UKHW051326070726
13610UKWH00014B/94

* 9 7 8 3 6 4 2 6 7 5 1 1 9 *